Positive
AGING

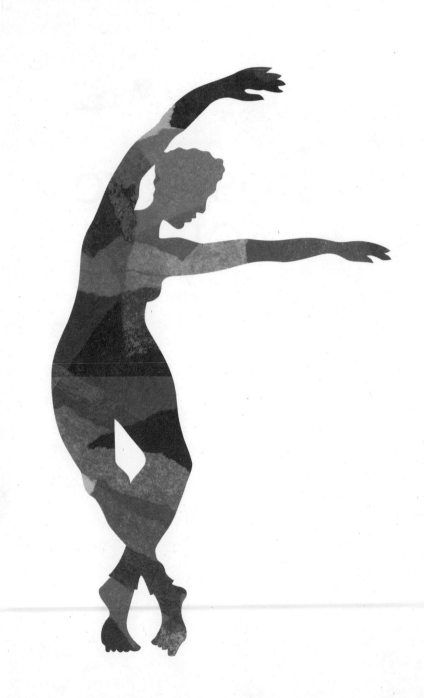

Positive
AGING

Every Woman's Quest
for Wisdom and Beauty

Karen Kaigler-Walker, Ph.D.

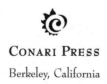

CONARI PRESS
Berkeley, California

Conari Press Books are distributed by Publishers Group West

Cover design: Suzanne Albertson
Cover illustration: Teresa Davis
Book design: Jennifer Brontsema
Author photo: Jerry De Wilde

ISBN: 1-57324-084-2

Library of Congress Cataloging-in-Publication Data
Kaigler-Walker, 1946–
    Positive aging: every woman's quest for wisdom and beauty / Karen Kaigler-Walker.
        p.   cm.
    Includes bibliographical references and index.
    ISBN 1-57324-084-2
    1. Middle aged women—United States—Psychology.   2. Middle aged women—
United States—Attitudes.   3. Self-esteem in women—United States.   4. Beauty,
Personal—United States—Psychological aspects.   I. Title.

HQ1059.5.U5K35   1997

305.244—dc21   97-1380

Printed in the United States of America on recycled paper.
10 9 8 7 6 5 4 3 2 1

For the Mothers:
Mary Homesley Kaigler
Lennie Wiseman Homesley
Lela Park Kaigler

For the Fathers:
Thomas A. Kaigler
Herbert Milton Homesley

For the Hero:
M. E. (Bud) Walker

Contents

Never a slave but in body,
now she has won freedom for her body, too.

—Damascius, *Epitaph* (Greek anthology)

The point is that the loss of soul connection,
loss of connection to our femininity, may be
the real cause of our anguished condition.

—Marion Woodman, *Conscious Femininity*

One

A Crack in the Mirror:
On Seeing Ourselves Age

A lump the size of Texas welled up in my throat as I read through the computer printouts from my latest research project. More than five hundred women from across the United States had answered questions on how they felt about their appearance, and their answers were making a single striking point: Those between the ages of thirty-five and fifty-five were troubled by how they looked. Not only were they troubled, but their dissatisfaction with their aging appearance left them feeling poorly about themselves in every other way.

I shared their distress. At age forty-four, I hardly needed statistics to verify that sometime around our fortieth birthday, we look into the mirror at sagging breasts, gathering wrinkles, or the silver in our once-raven hair and ask, "Why me?" and "What now?" Regardless of whether we are stay-at-home mothers, business tycoons, or professors, as women approach middle age the looking glass becomes a silent enemy that reminds us daily that we aren't the girls we used to be. Instead, the girl is being replaced by a woman who is no longer recognizable to us.

1

I, too, saw an aging stranger in my bathroom mirror. One morning I asked that foreign woman, "Who are you?" and stood there waiting for an answer—as though my body might shed some light on her masquerade.

To be sure, I wasn't alone. Everywhere I went—work, parties, seminars, even the library one afternoon—I heard the same grinding questions and perplexing uncertainties from women my age. Because I've researched women's appearance for the past twenty years, friends turned to me for help. But nothing had prepared me for the perplexity they—or I—felt.

After lo these many centuries of women growing older, one would hope that the bugs would be worked out by now! After all, although most of our foremothers lived shortened life spans, some *did* attain ripe old age. But because our death-denying society has so little appreciation of what it means to live past the twenties and thirties, we're left unprepared to move into our middle and later decades. As Maura Kelsea writes in *Women of the 14th Moon,* "Where, in our culture, do we have the expectation of becoming a Wise Woman? Who are our models?"

Even if we have expectations of aging in grace and wisdom, we have precious few socially acclaimed examples of how a venerated older woman might look. I recall a group of us sitting around a table, passing around a bottle of wine, and finally coming to the conclusion that regardless of what they accomplish, fifty-year-old women win society's acclaim only when they still look thirty-five. No standards exist for the attractive forty, fifty, sixty, or seventy year old who *actually* looks her age. It's no wonder physical aging is such an issue for us.

Aging and Loss

The quandary over our aging appearance looms large as we round the bend toward forty or fifty, because aging is treated the same as a deadly cancer by our culture—the blight that kills off our youthfulness. Madison

Avenue dictates that we defy age, the medical profession tries to cure it, and each year dozens of books hit the best-seller list that offer ways to live into our advanced decades as though we were still twenty.

Yet despite our efforts to ignore, defy, or cure it, the shadow of aging creeps up on us like a cloud passing over the sun as we reach thirty-five, forty-five, or fifty-five. And when it does—when we see our bodies age— we shudder.

In 1990, Ruth Hamel wrote in *American Demographics*: "The oldest baby boomers will turn 50 in 1996, and there's no indication that they'll expect or accept physical [aging]." Did *that* prophesy ever ring true! In our rage against aging, boomers spend more time, money, and energy than any previous generation on trying to hold back our ticking clock.

And why wouldn't we? Throughout our lives, we who are now in our forties and early fifties set the standards for the entire American culture in terms of lifestyle, values, and attitudes, including beauty and fashion. In our youth, high on the opiate of political vigor and youthful attractiveness and buoyed up by sheer numbers, we forged society's preoccupation with youth and beauty and established the nubile child-woman as an icon.

We came home from college, braless and swathed in army fatigues, to mothers who were less than eager to concede that the era of the cashmere sweater and little black dress was past. Yet soon, they, too, bared their forty-year-old knees and wore flat-chested shapeless dresses inspired by us, their daughters. By the 1970s, denim and fringe crowded Paris runways, and in the '80s we accustomed boardrooms to our chic, slim-hipped, skirted suits.

But now society's ideal female image doesn't reflect *us* anymore. Our aging looks no longer set the standard of beauty. Instead, we're dominated by it, shackled to an iron-clad norm of physical attractiveness that doesn't include gray hair, flabby chins, and ten extra pounds.

Since society believes that only youthful beauty will do, we're conditioned to think "old" when we first see milky traces of cellulite on our once-smooth thighs or the fine wrinkles around our eyes. And what does an old appearance say? It says we've lost our juice—our power, sexuality, and worth. Ironically, just when we reach the peak in our professions, earning capacity, mothering, and intellectual pursuits, our aging bodies appear to undermine our abilities and negate our rewards. Just when we are blossoming in every conceivable way, we're left feeling the bloom is off the rose.

How different the transition into menopause is from our journey into adolescence! We marched by the millions to Johnny Rivers, Petula Clark, the Beatles, and Simon and Garfunkel, who sang out about eagerly getting ready for an unknown tomorrow, of not knowing where we were going but bursting at the seams to get there. Today we hear no such marches. Instead, oldies music stations crank out reminders of the way it was, as all that is hip now passes us by. Magazines and talk shows offer up scores of talented, competent, energetic, and savvy women our age. Yet what snags our attention as we wend grocery baskets through the maze of tabloids on our way to the register is Oprah's diet, Cher's plastic surgery, and Hillary's haircut (there's even a web site where we can view all of her hairdos— more than 300 of them—since she became first lady).

If only our obsession with youthful beauty ended at the checkout line! But too often we concentrate on our changing looks to the exclusion of our other assets, just as we overlook those of the women in *People*. One day I asked my husband, Bud, if he'd noticed the changes in me, thinking of my shifting hipline and the chin that appeared to be leaving my face. "Yes," he answered, "you don't set goals and accomplish them anymore." It took several months for the full meaning of his response to sink in. At the time, I was so hopelessly ensnared in my "waning" appearance that I missed the point of his answer as surely as he missed the point of my question.

No, instead of focusing on the accomplishments in our lives, we pick up the phone and call Jenny Craig™ or visit cousin Bert the plastic surgeon, while our bookshelves groan under the weight of books on how to defy autumn's cycle through exercise, vitamins, and mind-over-body regimes that claim to keep us as fresh as our spring-green daughters.

The Inner Call

Our burgeoning bookshelves also attest to our need for self-discovery. In the late eighties, I read a blurb in *Writer's Market* that self-help and psychology markets would dry up by the mid-1990s. But, we who stand at the gates of middle age still surge into Barnes and Noble like birds to a feeding station seeking sustenance—hungering to reach in, evaluate our lives up to now, and come to terms with ourselves.

Psychologist Carl Jung maintained that our middle decades are indeed the time of reevaluating our lives, especially our ego's dependency on the external, material world with its focus on power and possessions. He believed that as we age we naturally shift our attention inward in search of what he called the *Self*. Much more than our conscious self, the Self resides deep within our unconscious and is the home of our soul, the place where the human meets the Divine. Jung spoke of our search for Self as the individuation process—coming to terms with who we are and what we're all about as ego selves so that we can connect to our greater Self and fulfill our larger, unique purpose during our middle and later decades.

In this, Jung put a very positive spin on aging that we never hear about in magazines or on talk radio. Yet his ideas about moving into our most creative and personally powerful years as we age into the second half of life more than explain why so many of us are drawn to self-examination as we near our middle birthdays.

Early in my forties I, too, wore a trail to the shelves marked "psychology" and "self-discovery." But instead of navigating the inner trail successfully, I became frustrated. Books, seminars, and tapes answered few of my questions about myself and offered minimal insight on the difficulties I was experiencing over my aging physique. Even my textbook knowledge about the workings of the psyche provided blessed little help. Instead, I felt split—body from soul—because no amount of reading seemed to quiet the hounds that bayed day and night about the diminishing worth of my appearance.

Epiphany

Early one cold Swiss morning I sat at the C. G. Jung Institüt in Zurich, warming my toes and waiting to hear author and analyst Kathrin Asper address our group. Little did I realize that during the next two days, she would provide the means for me to bridge the split between my appearance and Self.

As a way of explaining how and why people often fail to connect to their higher Selves, Dr. Asper reminded us of the Greek myth about Narcissus, the beautiful youth who fell in love with his reflection in a pool and starved to death because he couldn't bear to leave it. Like Narcissus, people can become so attached to their external lives—to power, turf, money, possessions, social standing, or image—that they fail to recognize and feed their soul and the Self withers and dies.

This was it! Like Narcissus, I was trapped by how I looked. As a woman, I believed my appearance *was* my power, as well as my turf, not to mention that how I looked reflected my social, professional, and economic value in the eyes of society. It would stand to reason that after decades of colluding with society's belief that a well-crafted appearance determines a woman's worth, I would look to my mirror to validate myself. Although I might not have wanted to admit it, anything I'd been or done other than how I looked was somehow secondary in my life. That's why I had lost sight of my accomplishments and abilities as I began to age!

Indeed, as I began to put two and two together, I realized that I wasn't alone in my appearance-related Narcissus complex. Countless women suffered from the same crippling syndrome—the friends who begged for answers as to why they felt so bad about themselves as they saw themselves age; the millions of midlife women nationwide who've recently felt the need for age-reduction surgery, making plastic surgery among the most lucrative branches of medicine today; and those of us who've vicariously felt the sting that an aging appearance brings as we wait to see if Joan Lunden really will lose her job as anchor of "Good Morning America" to a younger, more attractive woman, à la Jane Pauley.

Unfortunately, Narcissus' story doesn't end with his death, and neither does ours end with merely being trapped in the mirror by gray hair and age spots. According to legend, even after Narcissus dies and goes into the underworld, he continues to be mesmerized by his reflection—this time in the dark, brooding river Styx. Equating the Greek underworld with my inner realm, I realized that unless I did something different, my natural drive to connect with my Self would ever be thwarted by my dressing table mirror pulling me back to my obsession with my appearance. No wonder the self-discovery books and tapes offered no relief! I'd starved my Self and turned into a stationary little flower—a narcissus—who was incapable of navigating the inner journey that should form the basis of the second half of my life.

Little wonder the books on beauty and the jars of creams that were supposed to bolster my self-esteem also had failed in their promises. I could have stood at the mirror for the next ten years affirming how good I looked, as many books suggest, or I could have applied beauty potions until I was eighty, but nothing would have given me the Self-acceptance I craved. For in truth, what I yearned for couldn't be achieved superficially.

I'd certainly been correct in feeling split. My outer and inner selves were so separate that neither of them recognized the other's existence. I was caught in a Catch-22—unless I reached in and reconnected to my Self, I was incapable of truly loving myself and my body. Yet before I could successfully put my foot onto the inner trail I first had to untangle the choke hold of my socially dictated focus on appearance.

But how to break the grip? It's one thing to discover that I and thousands like me suffered from a vise that strangles our journey toward positive aging and the wholeness it brings. It's another to dismantle it.

Ancient Ways, Ancient Truths

Over the years as I began to explore this issue first with myself and then with hundreds of other women, I came to see that the first step in prying off the icy fingers of a youth-based standard is becoming aware of society's twisted notions about both female attractiveness and aging by tapping into a deeper truth about women's appearance and power. For believe me, the assumption that women have a lifelong need for peachy skin and a firm rear end is the by-product of a time when women were forced off the natural path of continued change, growth, and beauty throughout their *entire* life cycles.

Historically, the belief that youth and a fashionable look set the standard for female worth is quite recent. From the dawn of humankind until the decline of Crete (1400 B.C.) and until colonization in the Americas, beautiful, powerful women of all ages bore little relationship to their emaciated modern sisters. Fortunately, although we may not previously have been aware of this earlier era, it's not as hard as we might think to tap back into the mindset of that time. As Clarissa Pinkola Estés writes in *Women Who Run With the Wolves*, "A woman need not live as though she was born in 1000 B.C. Nevertheless, the old knowing is universal knowing, eternal and immortal learning, which will be as relevant five thousand years from now as it is today, and as it was five thousand years ago. It is archetypal knowing, and that kind of knowledge is timeless."

Like others who help women search for lost aspects of our feminine nature, I view fairy tales and myths as a means of cutting through recently distorted beliefs and delving into earlier truths. Although fairy tales, legends, and myths may seem mere children's stories, they only joined Mother Goose in the nursery bookcase early in the twentieth century.

Prior generations understood full well that these stories guide adults both in their daily lives and in communicating with the greater unknown. "A fairy tale holds the images of creation in the psyche," writes Jungian Lee Zahner-Roloff. "Unassailable in their rightness, in opposition to the human lived experience of daily events, they hold another way, another vision, another possibility."

Tales and myths hold other possibilities because they speak in metaphors—the symbolic language of the heart. Their imagery seeps into our deepest collective memory and stirs us profoundly. Since we're so used to living in our heads and viewing ourselves according to the dictates of society, our beleaguered bodies and parched souls are desperate for mythology's healing waters, for the essential truth such tales provide connects mind and heart and makes us whole.

Revisiting fairy tales holds special treasures for women, because we fare poorly by the sexist versions of western civilization's most potent stories. Disney and other purveyors of culture reduce young heroines to mere beautiful shells and older women to doddering fairy godmothers and wicked witches. Their versions of "Snow White," "Cinderella," and "Sleeping Beauty," in particular, demean us greatly. Reinterpreting older versions of these stories can allow us to reassess our culture's erroneous and dysfunctional assumptions about the original, sacred purposes of our aging bodies and their adornment, and reintroduces us to the authentic beauty of this stage in our lives.

The Heroine's Path

Tapping into ancient truths about female appearance is one thing, but actually reprogramming our opinions about how we look is something else again. Like the Sumerian goddess Inanna who was forced to shed her garments before she could enter the underworld and reunite with severed parts of herself, one by one, we must remove the old notions about aging that bar us from entering the gates to our souls. As Inanna discovered, the process is arduous, albeit it necessary and ultimately rewarding. Seven times as she traveled the underworld she had to give up a piece of her clothing and stoop low beneath a gate. At each gate she refused, demanding to be treated like the queen she was. But each time she finally backed down, and so she entered the underworld bowed and naked.

As I traversed the path to my Self, I often reeled under the pressure. Like Inanna, I demanded to be excused from giving up my old beliefs about my aging appearance. I had a secure position at my university, a good marriage, and more to do than I could say grace over. A little nip here and a tuck there would have given me back my former looks, and I could have forced my life to go on for a while more as it had for the past decades. But each time I wavered, a little voice from within reminded me that there was much in store for me if I persisted. Over and again, it assured me that as difficult as the journey seemed, if I wished to truly grow beautifully into the decades that awaited me, I must first strip myself naked of my former reliance on youthful, packaged beauty and walk on.

The First Step

I don't want to make the path to positive aging seem overly daunting. It isn't. If you're willing to accept two truths at this point, the rest will take care of itself as you move from one gate to the next.

First, your desire for beauty is innate; it comes from spirit, not from Seventh Avenue. What hamstrings us as we age isn't wanting to be beautiful, but society's erroneous notion that only the young are beautiful. Wanting to be beautiful is good, it's healthy—a gift from the Divine. So freeing yourself of society's "shoulds" regarding how you look and giving expression to your spirit-inspired, authentic appearance is the highest honor you can bestow on your Self.

Second, developing your authentic appearance has less to do with *what* you do to make yourself beautiful than *why* you do it. After all, women have been adorning themselves since before the dawn of history and have used every means available in doing so. Therefore, this isn't a how-to but a why-to book. And as you'll soon discover, there's a big difference.

So begin the journey to reconnect your body and soul via an authentic appearance confidently. You can do it! After all, as L'oréal's Preference™ ads suggest, "You're worth it."

My Appearance, My Self

The following exercise will help you discover the role your appearance plays in your life. For best results, read through and complete Part I first before you read and answer Part II. Get two clean sheets of paper and a pen, then take a few moments and relax your mind and body.

Part I – As fast as you can, write down as many words as you can think of that describe you. Write down *all* words that come to mind—the positive, negative, and in-between. The more words you write down the better. Keep writing until you cannot think of any more words, then set the paper aside.

Part II – Turn to the second sheet and make five columns. Label them "Roles," "Talents," "Personality," "Beliefs and Values," and "Appearance." Then put each word on your list from the first page into the appropriate category. Under "Roles" you might have words such as *mother* and *lawyer*. Under "Talents" list your abilities (artistic, good with numbers). "Personality Traits" will contain words such as *sincere* and *jealous*. In the fourth column, list your beliefs and values such as Jewish, love, or honor. Terms such as *brunette, overweight,* and *well-dressed* go in the appearance category.

Then look at all your columns. By comparing and contrasting the words in each category, you'll discover how you feel about yourself. Look at the length of each column. Do the words present a wide variety or a limited number of traits or abilities? How positive or negative are the words?

Don't be surprised if your appearance list runs long. After all, according to society, your appearance defines you. On the other hand, if this list is short or nonexistent, ask yourself why. In studying these lists you begin to develop an understanding of how you assess your appearance in comparison to your other traits, talents, and accomplishments. Refer back to your lists as you read on. They'll provide valuable insight into your relationship with your appearance.

*Our psychological being has been severed
from our biological selves for so long that we
are completely cut off from our true natures.*

—Elinor W. Gadon, *The Once and Future Goddess*

 Two

The Split:
Rending Body and Soul

There's no better way to begin the journey to connect body and soul than by revisiting an era that existed well before our modern attitudes about age and beauty took hold. There we find the most noted female trinity in mythology: Demeter, Kore—also known as Persephone—and Hecate, women who were spoken of long before even the Greeks, who made them famous.

The harvest goddess, Demeter, had a beautiful, young daughter, Kore, whom she loved very much. One fine day while Kore was out with friends, she found herself alone. As she reached down to pick a flower, a hole opened up in the earth through which Hades, the king of the underworld, came up. Grabbing the maiden, he pulled her down into his dark realm against her will to be his wife. Demeter frantically roamed the earth looking for Kore. During these days the earth remained unnourished, and the crops began to wither.

Though Demeter asked the other gods what they knew about Kore's disappearance, they refused to help her for fear of Zeus, who had looked the other way when Hades took the girl. Only when the crone-goddess of the underworld, Hecate, heard Demeter's cries and took pity on the grieving mother did Demeter learn of her daughter's fate.

In a fit of rage at Zeus' unwillingness to save Kore from rape, Demeter refused to water the earth until her daughter was returned to her; and the land suffered further. Seeing the plight of the earth and its people, the gods and goddesses pled with Zeus to free Kore (now married and known as Persephone). Fearing Demeter's power to decimate the earth, Zeus negotiated Persephone's release.

But because Persephone had eaten three pomegranate seeds while living with Hades, she was allowed to return to Demeter for only nine months each year. During the other three she lived as Hades' wife, reigning as queen of the underworld. For those months she was befriended by Hecate.

So for three-quarters of the year the earth is lush with fruit and grain. The other three months lie cold and barren, a reminder that Persephone has again left her mother and returned to the underworld and Hecate's care.

The story of Demeter's frantic search for Kore and the gray-haired goddess who befriends them speaks not of two-dimensional characters but of deeply seated archetypes—reoccurring figures in dreams and stories throughout history that touch us in a profound way. The three women represent three aspects of the Great Mother—the primal ancient female diety, often referred to as "Gaia"—and, as such, symbolize potent female figures in all of us who reside in our unconscious as the maiden, matron, and crone.

Although we might think of the maiden Kore as a young, sexual virgin, she actually represents a youthful, idyllic state of mind that can occur at any age, irrespective of our sexual experience. She's the childlike part of us that's lured off the path by pungently sweet flowers whose scent we can't resist. So we abandon our projects and abdicate responsibilities and merrily wander into places where we shouldn't be until we finally get into hot water. Then we're helpless until someone older and wiser (or some older and wiser aspect of ourselves) comes to our rescue.

Mythologist Robert Graves describes the matron, Demeter, as "a gentle soul," given to kindness—not common among Greek goddesses who were known more for hot tempers and nothing short of overkill when it came to meting out punishment. Yet Demeter was loving, even to the point in another myth of lessening the punishment of Erysichthon, the only man she ever cursed. That she withheld rain when she lost Kore can't be viewed as selfish, but as feminine finesse. For what mother wouldn't play her highest card to win back a daughter who'd been kidnapped and raped?

The crone goddess Hecate is the least remembered of the three. Indeed, my first exposure to this story when I was in the second grade made no mention of Hecate at all. This oversight plays right into modern western culture's beliefs about the invisibility of older women, witnessed again more recently by the omission of Hecate from most of the popular goddess books. Yet, were it not for Hecate, Demeter would have roamed the earth withholding rain until choking dust blew away the last wisp of grain. And it is Hecate who befriends and ministers to Persephone during her annual wintry return to the underworld. She's so necessary to the maiden that in some versions of the myth, Hecate walks before and behind Persephone in spirit form while Persephone is on the earth with Demeter.

Legend also holds that Hecate is so potent that Zeus gives her free rein to bestow or withhold gifts to travelers who come to the dark subterranean crossroads where she stands with her hounds and torch. Yet she is much more than a mere guide to the underworld. Because Hecate's realm is the netherworld between life and death, that murky arc in the circle of life where transformation and regeneration occur before rebirth can take place, she is mighty, abundant, wise, and farsighted—vastly familiar with the ways and means of spirit.

The Ancient Crone

While society may now view the crone as a witch, in pre-Judeo/Christian eras she bore no resemblance whatsoever to Webster's modern definition of "a withered old woman." Indeed in that time which Joseph Campbell spoke of as, "below the ultimate horizon of humanity," older women like Hecate were a power to be reckoned with.

That's because in societies dating from the Ice Age to 1100 B.C. in the Old World and until colonization in the Americas, age was a valuable and rare commodity. The blood—the elixir of life—she no longer shed monthly was believed to remain in her womb and empower her in other ways. So as a woman matured past menopause, she grew in stature until, in advanced age, she was venerated.

I've heard it argued that older women were held in high esteem simply because so few women lived past their second or third decades. But this argument simply doesn't hold water. If primitive women past childbearing years had been venerated for nothing more than longevity, the scarcity of food soon would have overshadowed their value to the clan and caused widespread geriatric euthanasia. Yet, no evidence exists for this in the earliest societies. No, the era of expendable village grandmothers came much later. During this period of prehistory, older women were the glue that held clans together.

Like Hecate, older women ministered to younger women—those still in their budding and blooming cycles—and sustained the tribe and healed the sick through their knowledge about growing grain and gathering medicinal herbs. Too, elder clanswomen assumed the role of midwife— helping others both give birth and die. For who but the experienced and wizened crone would know so much about the arc in the circle of life which connects death and birth?

In their advanced years, women became the keepers of the sacred stories and tenders of the ancestral spirits. Thus they assumed the mighty role of tribal link between human and supernatural. The spiritual counterparts of these gray-haired high priestesses were known throughout the primal world as Hecate, Sophia, Q're, Edda, and Old Spider Woman, among hundreds of other goddesses whose names meant wisdom, power, mother of truth, intelligence, and prophecy.

Sacred Sexuality

Early on, powerful female goddesses also ruled over human sexuality. Sex was seen as neither sinfully erotic nor solely linked with fertility but one and the same as nature's most potent force—the powerful, creative feminine. So, for example, Aphrodite was much more than the goddess of romantic love and beauty. She blessed the people with sculpture, poetry, and music, as well as sensuality and sexuality. Demeter was the quintessential earth mother, fruitful, yes, but also powerful and able to accomplish great things. Hecate not only ministered to the young Persephone, but she was the patron goddess of abundance and eloquence—that which is reaped from using talents.

And it wasn't only the goddesses who were potent. In various societies throughout the ancient world, including many Native American tribes, postmenopausal women's sexual knowledge and skill were so respected that the young men were sent to them for instruction, including hands-on experience, before marriage.

It stands to reason, therefore, that our earliest foremother's bodies were full of their own worth and bursting with positive sexual/creative energy. We can still feel this unabashed eroticism exuding from ancient clay sculptures and cave paintings that even after all these centuries seem too hot to handle.

Adorned in Spirit

Our foremothers' world abounded with spirit. And nowhere was spirit more evident than in women's appearance. Ancient women adorned themselves as an act of worship, one that honored their bodies as temples of spirit in the fullest sense of the metaphor. Skin and bark wraps, waist strings, paint, tattoos, scars, or whatever else was worn declared the oneness of mind, body, and soul with the great universal power that played such a pivotal role in the life of the clan.

Even preparing clothing and others' adornment was women's sacred work. Before the mists of recorded history, yarn from which cloth was woven symbolized the thread of life—the umbilical cord that binds child to mother, the link between the conscious and unconscious, the strand between heaven and earth. As such, yarn was *wakan*—holy and powerful female stuff. Indeed, women's hair, the original yarn, still holds a mystical aura, shining with the light of the powerful properties of the ancient feminine. And like the ancient feminine, it continues to grow. It may be singed, cropped, ripped out, or shaved off, but it comes back—beautiful, natural, and shining.

Not only was yarn sacred, but so was the cloth made from it. According to southwestern Native American legend, Great Spirit's first gift to humans was cloth-making. Other early stories from around the globe also spoke of sacred weaving. Athena wove; so did the Sumerian goddess Uttu. The goddess Queen Goya taught Incan women how to weave cotton and wool. Old Norse legend held that humans wove their destiny into cloth. And according to the Greeks, Penelope charted her own course by weaving at her loom by day and rending warp from weft at night to stave off the suitors who would come for her should she have finished. Not too far away, the returning Ulysses stored his treasures in the moist cave of the Naiads, weavers of garments the color of blood—life itself. "In the ancient world," writes Tivka Frymer-Kensky in *In the Wake of the Goddess:*

Women, Culture, and the Biblical Transformation of Pagan Myth, "women were often depicted as holding a hand-spindle and a whorl, the characteristic symbol of femininity."

Clothing and household goods made from cloth were holy also. Navajo women wove rugs that were products of mind, body, and soul. The numinous yarn linked the sheep who gave the wool, the mind and hand of the weaver, and the greater all in all; thus their rugs affirmed the holy in vivid hues and sacred motifs. Half a world away and a millennium earlier, women of ancient Athens spent nine months each year sewing a *peplos* (short dress) for the goddess Athena.

So early human adornment, be it with aprons, paint, arm bands, or feathers, symbolized the very fabric of existence and the connection to spirit. But it had social meaning as well. What a woman wore stated publicly who she was by showing her place within her family, her marital status, her age, and any and all other pertinent information about her. Too, shells she plaited in her hair or paint she brushed on her body linked her with her female heritage, because at each stage of her life she wore the same garb as had her mother, grandmother, and as many great-greats as could be remembered from out of the foggy past. In this way, a woman was assured of who she was and of the lofty part she played in her community.

Color also translated into mystical symbolism. Red was the color of the matron—Demeter in the fullness of her years. Black was the color of the powerful crone in Old Europe. In the Old World white symbolized the maiden, while among northern Native Americans and Eskimos it was worn by elder clanswomen. Regardless of whether age was symbolized by black or white, however, the colors were donned as badges of honor by women who had lived long, well, and wise.

Beyond red, black, and white, other colors imbued the wearer with special powers or invoked the gods and goddesses. Nature's green was sacred to Venus and the blue of the sky to Jupiter and Juno. Plains Indian mothers gave newborns a personal power color in addition to a name.

Special colors and adornment also marked the sacredness of ceremonies as well as a woman's emotional bond with members of her clan, both living and dead.

Our foremothers didn't paint, pierce, and dress to acknowledge oneness with spirit just for special occasions. Since work ensured life, life's work was deemed hallowed. Still today, the Cebecar Indians of Costa Rica have no word for ceremony because all of life is viewed as a ceremony. So early on, that which was worn for gathering berries for hungry bellies was no more or less sacred than that donned for birth, marriage, and death.

The older woman's adornment was the same as her goddess counterpart, whose images were etched in stone, molded in clay, and painted on the walls of caves throughout the primeval world. Village grandmothers proudly wore the sacred vestments of the goddess, be she Scandinavia's Edda or Spider Grandmother of the New World.

It's important to note that our earliest foremothers had no notion of fashion as we think of it today, for they had no concept of wearing styles because they were new and popular. Similarly, they didn't wear status symbols in the modern sense. Inasmuch as humans were viewed as being one with nature, taking her bounty was an act of sharing rather than of conquest. So wrapping one's naked body in the skin of a recent kill paid homage to the animal who sacrificed its life so that the clan could survive. Wearing the skin assured that the spirit of the animal would return to guide upcoming hunts.

Women accrued status not in furs and jewels and youthfully thin bodies but by having children early in life and through serving the community in wisdom and spirit after menopause. Silver in a mature woman's hair symbolized her connection with her spirit-mother, the moon, and the rest of her countenance also was lauded as that of a sage and necessary member of the clan. Thus her aging body was honored as a temple.

Severed Image

What happened? How did society get from viewing the woman at midlife as perched to come into her spiritual own, a valuable and honored figure, to seeing middle-aged bodies as needing tummy tucks?

It wasn't an overnight process. Just how the mirror seduced us took well over six millennia and completely upended the social order, religious structure, and politico/economic base of the earliest human societies. Beginning around 4300 B.C., marauding bands of Kurgan, Aryan, Hittite, Mittani, Luwian, Achaean, Dorian, and Hebrew warriors swept through the ancient cradles of civilization. Crete, the last and most highly developed Old World society, collapsed in 1100 B.C. Then beginning again in A.D. 1492, European colonizers took about four hundred years to subdue the indigenous peoples of the Americas. In all of these conquerors' wakes, the sacred link between women's body and soul was severed, thus setting up the conditions that led us to where we are today.

The nomadic warriors were different from the older societies in almost every way, for their social order hinged on a rigid, male-dominated, social hierarchy rather than on the primal feminine concept of equality. As time progressed and the new model began to dominate, linear, hierarchical thinking replaced intuition as the chief means of gaining knowledge. The belief that men not only had the right but the duty to conquer the land and its creatures supplanted the older concept of being in partnership with nature, and a man's worth became the amount of land, animals, and gold he owned. Science became divorced from spirit, and technology was crowned king.

The ancient belief in women's special kinship with spirit stuck in the craw of this new order like a chicken bone. Over time, in the name of jealous, demanding, and often monotheistic male gods, women's vaulted position as high priestess was stripped from them as men assumed the sole right to the priesthood.

Early on, Christianity appeared to offer hope that women would again be recognized as conduits of spirit. Instead, however, Christianity soon incorporated Saint Paul's misogynist views rather than honoring the feminine as did Saint John and the Gnostics, and by the early Middle Ages, theologians presumed that women were hopeless sinners with no souls at all.

Branding women as infidels was merely the first cut. As centuries passed, older women were barred from the diverse tasks they had performed in earlier societies, as male priests and chieftains co-opted their former roles and came to serve as teachers, healers, and craft-makers, thereby robbing women of the rich, diverse growth and contribution formerly associated with their middle and later decades.

The only aspect of womanhood that the patriarchs could not rout was women's ability to conceive and bear children, so they sought to control it. Thus women retained only one acceptable function—to produce children, specifically, male heirs. This legacy carried forward into the early twentieth century as affirmed by German spokesperson of the Catholic working class, Franz Hitze, who wrote that woman's only rightful places were the *Küche* (kitchen), *Keller* (cellar), and *Kleiderschrank* (closet).

Casting out all but the single function of cloistered mother not only restricted women's activities, but it collapsed the female life cycle of maiden, matron, and crone. No wonder the youthful female body came to have so much cultural value! If a woman's sole job was to procreate, being young and looking good was vital to her success.

The most popular fairy tale heroines speak of the esteem now accorded to nubile maidens. Like middle-aged female movie stars, Demeter and Hecate no longer hold center stage, as young and innocent girls get the lead roles. The most graphic fairy tale symbol of the collapsed life cycle is Snow White, with her white (maiden) skin, blood-red (matron) lips, and hair as black as ebony (crone).

Given that the full measure of women's worth rested in their fertile years, the menopausal woman became superfluous. Unable to provide the much-prized offspring, she represented a financial drain to the medieval church. Poor widows took up precious financial resources, yet had little to contribute back. If wealthy, an older woman stood to inherit valuable land, depriving it from either the church or her male heirs.

Cursed Legacy

An even greater affront than a postmenopausal woman's drain on church coffers, however, was the dormant power resting in her unconscious—a throwback to the days when postmenopausal women shifted from matrons to mighty crones. While by the Middle Ages women may have been reduced to little more than providers of sex and male heirs, their innate feminine qualities couldn't be eradicated by decree. Deep within, the midlife women still knew too much, spoke too much truth, and carried too much power. Despite the church, they continued to illicitly practice herbal healing and midwifery as well as display their natural affinity for animals, trees, and other things of the land. But even more insidious to the church fathers, these women still retained knowledge of the time when older women accessed spirit directly rather than going through an intermediary male clergy.

Eventually elderwomen who followed the ancient ways were castigated from the pulpit and town hall where they were called old wags, hags, and lunatics. Ironically, these degrading epithets that were hurled at village grandmothers were degenerated cognates of ancient words of praise for the crone goddesses—hag came from *hagia,* meaning holy woman; *luna* referred to an older woman's connection with the moon; and the word *crone,* which came from the same root word as crown, is still so despised and misunderstood that one of my friends recently asked me to quit using it around her.

Public tongue lashings, however, were mild in comparison to the ultimate fate of many women. From the thirteenth through the seventeenth centuries, somewhere between five and nine million women in Europe and the American colonies, most of whom were older and/or childless, were labeled as witches for their heretical beliefs and practice of herbal medicine and midwifery. Then they were slain in an effort to save their souls as well as those of the surviving villagers.

The torture and death of these millions of innocent older women burned deep into our collective unconscious. No wonder we reel in terror at the onslaught of middle age. The message about aging that our unconscious received from those centuries of anguish is far more sinister and foreboding than anything from the pen of Stephen King.

Lust of the Eye

By this point in history, it appears that women were left with little other than the skin over their bones. But even this outer covering was far from overlooked, as the female body became the battleground on which the clergy fought the war against the feminine. Youthful female beauty was deemed the primary tool by which the devil snared honest men, while the naturally aged look of the older woman was proof positive that the devil had won.

Demeter's once mighty red became the color of the prostitute—the hedonistic and lustful woman who operated outside society's rigid code of conduct for goodly (godly) women. These women, who dared use their own bodies (and presumably minds) for their own purposes and desires, were ostracized, as was exemplified when Hester Prynne was sentenced to wear the scarlet letter.

But of course, even after centuries of tirades against it, the desire for female beauty couldn't be routed, either from men who craved it or from the women who wanted to look attractive. The love of beauty is too intrinsic. Rather, it came to be that female beauty, like female sexuality, was acceptable only *if* and *when* it was controlled by men. In support of this, medieval theologian Thomas Aquinas wrote that it was good for women to adorn themselves in order to cultivate the love of their husbands, ". . . in that they lighten the fatigue of our labors." So throughout her lifetime, a woman's beauty remained the property of her father, brother, uncle, husband, and priest lest she dare use it for her own sexual or self-expressive desires.

Still today, as we struggle to free ourselves from the legacy handed down by the fathers of western society, we're reminded time after time in fairy tales the extent to which female beauty is male-dominated— Sleeping Beauty's father sequestered her; asexual male dwarfs sheltered Snow White and a male bear protected the sisters in the story of "Snow White and Briar Rose"; and young and beautiful queens, such as the "Handless Maiden," were left with mothers-in-law or faithful servants as husbands rode off to war. Indeed, in all my research, I've yet to come across a fairy tale in which a man dies or goes off and leaves an attractive, young wife to fend for herself. Such story patterns both reveal and reinforce our rigid assumptions.

Western culture so thoroughly adopted the belief that the only virtuous purpose of female attractiveness is to assist a woman in her role of wife and mother that post-Victorian costume historian James Laver theorized that women's desire for adornment *originated* from our innate need to attract the opposite sex. He surmised that dependent primitive females *had* to decorate themselves to attract a mate and keep him sexually satisfied so that he would feed and protect her and her children. Laver called his theory the Principle of Seduction.

The theory seemed sound. Given a woman's position in late-nineteenth and early-twentieth-century English society, attracting and keeping a husband *was* vital to her welfare. On her own she had no social standing, no property, and no respectability, so it was reasonable to assume that maintaining a sexually alluring appearance was paramount.

Not surprisingly, Laver never mentioned the purpose of women's adornment past their childbearing years. Since he developed his theory on the heels of the most sexually repressive era in modern history and on the eve of western culture's budding love affair with youth, he had no reason to assume that attractiveness was necessary after menopause.

Indeed, midlife women's appearance had undergone quite a transformation. Whereas in the earliest societies they had gaily adorned themselves in celebration of their upcoming cronehood, middle-aged women under patriarchy were most often draped in somber tones that hid them. They were relegated to drab, sexless, insipid styles in expectation that they would merely evaporate into the confines of their own hearths. Black, once the mighty color of Hecate, shrouded the widow—the woman who had neither purpose nor position because she lacked a husband. Woe be it to the widow who donned finery and acted as though she was anything but dead to life. Remember widowed Scarlet O'Hara dancing with Rhett Butler? She set tongues to wagging all over Georgia.

In fairy tales, the black-clad older woman fell into infamy as the wicked stepmother (the other mother), Baba Yaga, sorceress, enchantress, and witch. And it's no accident that the vast majority of these fairy tale crones were portrayed as ugly—snaggle-toothed and wart-covered—for along with the social denigration of the older woman came a vilification of the natural changes in her body. Barbara Walker, symbologist and author of *The Crone: Woman of Age, Wisdom, and Power,* writes, "It became the conventional opinion that all old women were ugly. The gray-haired high priestesses, once respected tribal matriarchs of pre-Christian Europe, were transformed by the newly dominant patriarchy into minions of the devil." So the Brothers Grimm painted the witch in "Jorinda and Joringea" as "a crooked old woman, yellow and lean, with large red eyes and a hooked nose, the point of which reached to her chin." To be sure, these are nothing more than exaggerated features of advanced age, and equating them with evil forges a powerful link in our subconscious between aging and sinfulness.

Walker writes further, "Patriarchal society often views physical ugliness as the worst of sins in a female, overriding all compensatory qualities of virtue, kindness, or intelligence, because these qualities are more or less irrelevant in a sex object. Ugliness is forgivable in men, but not in women. Consequently and conversely, ugliness is also attributed to any female who might be labeled sinful." No wonder we fear aging like the plague. According to the culture in which every one of us was born and raised, we sin against society as our bodies age through their natural cycle, and the effect of these deeply held unconscious attitudes on our individual psyches cannot be discounted.

The Birth of Fashion

Down through the centuries, however, despite the pyre, the pulpit, and the veil, women of all ages remained firm in their desire to make themselves beautiful. Although severed consciously from the original purpose of their adornment—the honoring of the connection between body and soul and between Self and all—they retained their inborn need to express themselves with cloth and paint on the canvas of their bodies. This craving for self-expression, coupled with the fact that little else in the way of entertainment or education was available to women, made the pursuit of fashion a full-time career for many women beginning in the Middle Ages.

Fashion took root in the thirteenth century in far-flung medieval manors and reached a zenith in the high Renaissance, a time when women owned virtually nothing, not even their own clothing. Instead, the bodies of wives and daughters served as mannequins for men, for a comely attired set of females defined a man's coffers and assured his place in the social hierarchy the same as owning a stable of fine horses.

During this time, Renaissance women of noble birth and the daughters of the newly moneyed bourgeoisie turned their full attention to outward finery. Chic Este and DeMedici women set the style throughout Europe. And the rest, as they say, is history. Women's appearance degenerated into a symbol of domination over the lower classes by the rich and powerful, and fine clothes and jewelry translated into the measure of female value.

As the original symbolism of women's adornment was turned on end, wanting to look fashionable became the *raison d'être* for adorning ourselves. What once bespoke of nurturance, healing, oneness with nature, harmony, wisdom, and spirit now stood for wealth, elitism, us versus them, and the worship of the new for its own sake. In the wake of the shift, women's appearance became little more than walking sign-boards of their families' social position and economic power.

At the end of the nineteenth century, for example, starched, white, pleated, and tucked linen dresses announced publicly that the women who wore them could afford to hire other women to keep their garments clean and pressed. Corsets rendered upper-class women unable to bend or even breathe, a sure sign that they didn't do physical labor—not even in their own homes. Today, we may be freer to take on more responsibilities, but designer logos and labels are so important to our feelings of Self that we wear them on the *outside* of our clothing so that others can't miss seeing our worth.

So, although we wend our way into a new millennium, things haven't changed as much for women as we might like to think. We're still entrapped in an appearance snare that was set centuries ago.

Body Loathing

This very brief overview of the past 10,000 years establishes the context for understanding the deep-seated cultural reasons why we women are so identified with our appearance and fearful of aging. Recent critiques of the fashion industry, such as *The Beauty Myth,* explain the form our obsession takes, but, as I've tried to indicate, the psychological roots of the problem go much deeper. We must, therefore, go deeper in quest of a solution.

Due to centuries of training, instead of conceiving of our bodies as integrated, living, breathing, spirit-filled entities that shift in purpose and appearance as we age, society expects us to treat them like commodities. And since we've been programmed to believe that our body is our most worthy commodity, we learn at an early age to trade on it in the marriage, business, and social markets the same as we might trade on cattle or grain futures. As such, when our body looks the way it "should" it is okay; we like our body. But when it doesn't, we loathe it: It's too tall, too fat, too lumpy, or too flat-chested. You name it and some woman has complained about it.

Although we negatively evaluate our body throughout our lives, as we age into our mid-decades, we tend to turn on it like an animal who gnaws at a paw that's caught in a trap. Unfortunately, too often, hating our body ultimately turns into self-mutilation. We may not like the ideas that remaking our body in the name of youthfulness through plastic surgery, continuing to smoke so that we won't gain weight, and strenuously dieting to where we have no fat in which to store life-sustaining minerals and vitamins mortify the flesh, but they *do*.

Indeed, when it comes to the injury we inflict as a result of our fear of aging, we often play out the ever-popular theme in fairy tales of the step-mother plotting to kill the maiden. We don't have to apply scientific measures to test our body's need for love and the devastation to our soul when it isn't received. Just visit any city kennel where animals are kept, fed, and watered but not really loved or nurtured, and you can't help but notice the spiritless look in the eyes that warily stare at you from the back of cages.

I also see that same vacant stare in the eyes of middle-aged and older women who aren't able to revere their bodies as temples of spirit. Although the skin on their faces may be as tight as a newly made bed and their bodies as fat-free as a super-model's, their eyes betray them. For as their eyes aged past the glow of maidenhood, they haven't been set aflame with the fire of real womanhood.

I'm reminded of bumping into a fifty-something business acquaintance of my husband's at a party. The man's wife looked as if she'd just been slapped.

"Oh, don't mind Paula," the husband boomed out, "she's just had a little liposuction. Soon she'll be back to being 'my little Paula' again."

"Yes, *your* little Paula," I thought.

The wounds we inflict when we carve away unwanted pieces of flesh, stand in front of the mirror and silently yell at our bodies in disgust, or starve in the names of fashion and youth, don't heal. Our lack of love registers deep into every cell. It invades our psyches like an evil stepmother, further fueling our feelings of unworthiness and eating away our self-esteem like a cancer.

Merely becoming aware of the pitfalls of midlife body loathing, however, won't help us shake it. The twisted attitudes about women's worth are far too entrenched in every nook and cranny of our psyches for that. Unless we consciously dig down to their roots, rout them out, and change our ways, we'll continue to hate our aging bodies—and ourselves—as we peer into the looking glass each morning and ask "Who's the fairest?"

Says Who?

It's one thing to discover that beliefs about our aging bodies are recent cultural lies, but it's another to change our attitudes about how we look. The following will help you analyze where some of your negative ideas originated and set the stage for you to send them packing.

If you listen to a group of women talk, you'll hear one woman complain about her square hips, another about drooping eyelids, and the third about a crapey neck. Given that all our bodies age similarly, you'd think we'd be concerned about what is happening to our various body parts equally. But we aren't.

For example, I don't view the cottage cheese on my thighs as any big deal, but I absolutely detest the flab on my upper arms. Why? Because as a child I heard the older women in my mother's family complain about their large upper arms. In other words, I was programmed to dislike my middle-aged arm flab long before I hit forty. Oh, my grandmother and her sisters had their share of cellulite! But bumpy thighs weren't a topic of discussion during those Sunday afternoons when they sat in the back room and talked about women things.

Take a few minutes and remember back to how you were conditioned to zero in on certain parts of your body, as I was. What did your mother dislike about her body? Your grandmothers? Your aunts? What are the assumptions about the way women in your family age? Your insight will disclose a pattern of body loathing that you're programmed to repeat unless you break the cycle. For just as we learn from our families what to value and devalue in other aspects of our lives, we're conditioned by them to age physically with certain built-in biases and expectations.

*Women who have learned to bank on their beauty
and who identify themselves with it find the aging
process unusually difficult because they see themselves losing everything they value and they believe
is of value in them. This is indeed a tragedy.*

—Dr. Joyce Brothers, *Los Angeles Times*

➤ Three

Motherless: Youthworship and Midlife Alienation

The demise of the feminine in the world certainly left us in a lose/lose situation when it comes to our aging bodies. And as with any loss, we must
first assess the damage before we can put ourselves right again.

In bygone days when such a mighty task lay ahead, a wise old grandmother would tell a story from which instruction would surface. I always
knew a magical story was forthcoming when my granny sat down, took off
her glasses, wiped them clean on the hem of her cotton house dress, and
said, "Well, let me see . . . *Once upon a time* . . ."

. . . *in a land not so far away, the wife of a wealthy man lay dying. She called
her young daughter to her and told the girl that if she stayed good and pious, God
would take care of her. The mother vowed that she would look down on the little girl
from heaven and remain nearby. After her mother died, the child went to her grave*

each day and wept, and she stayed good and pious. The snow laid a white blanket over the grave, and, when the spring sun had melted it away, the man had taken another wife.

The new wife had two daughters of her own. And although they were fair of face, their hearts were evil. They treated the child badly and forbid her to sit in the parlor. Instead, they took the girl's pretty clothes and slippers, gave her a gray bedgown and wooden shoes to wear, and banished her to the kitchen where she worked by day and slept among the ashes at night. Soon, her face and gown were covered with soot, so they called her Cinderella.

Here we have the fairy tale we loved to read again and again as children because it reassured us that although we might feel like soot-covered outcasts, we really were beautiful princesses just waiting to be discovered. But Cinderella's story about the nature of female beauty isn't limited to little girls; it's every bit as relevant today as it was when we were six. For in our middle decades we again search for beauty while feeling like strangers in our own bodies. And it is the Cinderella in us—the uncontaminated knowledge that we are innately good and that our bodies are temples of our souls—that we quest for. But before we can rediscover the authentic beauty that dwells within us and bring it into our life and allow it to help us in our upcoming season, like Cinderella we must work through the trials that beset us.

Death of the Mother

When the story opens, we meet a nameless young mother identified only as the wife of a rich man. In contrast to powerful Demeter, we hardly recognize this mother's importance to the story because she soon dies. But the mother's short role is far from insignificant.

In a mythic sense, the mother's early death symbolizes the demise of the ancient feminine by the early Middle Ages, when this version of Cinderella's story emerged. Her death reminds us that the goodly woman's role now was merely to bear offspring. By dying, the mother seals her goodness, for she has "done her job" and won't face the possible evil that maturity might bring.

It's not just Cinderella's mother who dies young and anonymously. Snow White and Vassalisa the Beautiful are similarly orphaned. In other stories, such as "Sleeping Beauty" and "Rapunzel," the mother doesn't die but is ineffective when her daughter is threatened. In each of these stories, the fairy tale mother is barred from her full Demeter role—grooming her daughter for adulthood, helping her through tough times, being there to answer questions about what it's like to be a woman, helping her flesh out her feminine roles—to say nothing of later taking Hecate's role and helping her daughter to develop her soul.

The only motherly advice Cinderella's mother imparts before she dies is when she asks Cinderella to remain good and pious. She promises that if Cinderella remains so, God will protect her and she will stay near by her.

Yet the mother's promise seems to fail. For despite following her mother's advice, Cinderella, like the earlier Persephone, finds herself in a terrible situation. Then she, too, falls to the care of an older woman. But the stepmother's interest in Cinderella differs in every way from Hecate's loving concern for Persephone.

Although we're no longer maidens, culturally we're like Cinderella—orphaned little girls who have no mother to teach us how to be whole women. For regardless of the individual mothering we received, the death of the Great Mother left us bereft of Her nurturing, especially as we enter our middle and later decades. For even if our mother lives to a ripe old age, she's probably ill-equipped to teach us the full scope of what it means to be either a maiden just ready to bloom or a matron on the verge of cronehood. She wasn't taught by her mother, and neither were our grandmothers taught by their mothers for as many generations back as we can count. Without proper mothering, we, too, find ourselves left in the hands of a stepmother.

The Wicked Stepmother

The fairy tale stepmother is the archetype of the split-off parts of the Great Crone that society fears most, for she inherited Hecate's knowledge of death and dying, as well as her might. But the stepmother failed to retain Hecate's understanding of rebirth, her ability to face the crossroads of life with insight, her ability to help bestow abundance and eloquence, and her love-based judgment regarding how to wield power. Without this balance, the stepmother is decay without regeneration, dark without light, and power without prudence. No wonder western society came to fear her and looked to youth as the repository of all that is good.

But the stepmother can't be done away with simply because we fear her evil, for archetypes can't be killed. They are powerful parts of us that must somehow be integrated into our psyches so that we can be whole. But because we haven't been taught to acknowledge and embrace this part of ourselves, we try to escape from her by shunning her to the backroom of our psyches.

Yet, that's just the way the stepmother likes it. By denying her existence, we free her to use every trick in the book to keep us from fulfilling the promise that is within us, thus wreaking havoc on our souls. In this, she plays a key role in our appearance-based narcissus complex. For just as Cinderella's mother's goodness and piety were passed along to Cinderella, the stepmother's vileness is the legacy of the stepsisters who throw Cinderella out of the parlor. Like them, we try to keep that part of us who knows the ancient truth about the purpose of our midlife and the role authentic appearance plays in it buried in our unconscious. In so doing, we allow the offspring of the evil stepmother to rule our egos.

The Lure of the Parlor

The parlor is the place in the home where we entertain outsiders, and it symbolizes the social arena wherein we interact with other people. After these many centuries of society valuing women primarily because of our public image, our ego is like Cinderella's stepsisters who view the parlor as their exclusive turf—especially when it comes to Cinderella. They don't consider Cinderella as their kin—as being part of them—so they refuse to have anything to do with the little waif. Similarly, after years of being unaware of that part of our Self which knows about authentic beauty, our ego fails to recognize it as being part of us. All our ego knows is that we've been judged by our parlor appearance since before we can remember, and that it feels like the only thing that gives us worth.

Needless to say, when our egos first encounter the orphaned child in us who knows the truth about authentic appearance, we, like the stepsisters, refuse to acknowledge her. I'm reminded of one of my closest friends who yelled in frustration when I first began to question our dependence on standardized, youthful beauty, "And just what are we *supposed* to do, grow gray hair down to our waists and wear muu-muus?" The answer is an emphatic no in her case, for that look wouldn't be reflective of her Self. But my friend wasn't yet ready to hear about positive aging. Instead, she derided the dirty little scullery maid who held the kernel of truth.

Yet there is more to banishing Cinderella than merely pitching out an uncomfortable reminder that authentic appearance is linked with the Self rather than Seventh Avenue. For although the stepsisters do the dirty work of sending Cinderella from the parlor, we must remember that they are the offspring of the stepmother who casts her evil through their actions. Likewise, our internal stepmother keeps our ego and Self apart so that she can work her evil.

Theologians, philosophers, and storytellers have long known that evil easily entices us with the very things we think we want, tricking us into its snare through our vanities. And, although the stepsisters may not know of their kinship with the child who holds the key to spirit-based, authentic beauty, the stepmother surely does. So as long as our Cinderella is held aside, we won't discover that our desire to adorn ourselves has to do with anything but the parlor. Our ego will continue to align with the well-dressed stepsisters who dance only to society's fashion tune.

As we age, the stepmother bumps up her effort to keep us focused on the parlor, for this is the time we'd otherwise appropriately turn in toward ourself. But the savvy old girl knows the prophets of old were correct in that we cannot follow two masters at the same time. By cunningly using our fear of aging to keep us busy maintaining a youthful appearance, she ensures that we shun the urge to reconnect us with our loving Self. And her trick works.

Her treachery results in a self-fulfilling prophecy. For when we make life denying choices in the name of packaged beauty rather than turn in and learn of the Self's promise for a meaningful, fruitful second half, we suffer spiritual death. We keep our Cinderella in the kitchen, continue to view aging as negative, and the regeneration that should follow the natural demise of our early years fails to take place. Thus the dreaded stepmother wins in the end.

The Kitchen

The kitchen where Cinderella was banished was the least desirable room in the feudal manor, often built underground or separate from the main house altogether so that cooking odors couldn't seep into the living quarters. The scullery maid was the lowest of the low, too dirty to keep company even with other household help, much less the family.

In the story the kitchen represents our unconscious, the deep ocean of images and memories of thousands of lifetimes and as many years, which undergird the human psyche. Like good and pious Cinderella who was stripped of her pretty clothes and forced into the kitchen, the orphan who

knows the truth about positive aging sits among the ashes in our unconscious and suffers for lack of the realization of who she really is.

But now that the child of the loving Mother has been discovered, we
cannot shut her away so easily. We're like the heroine in Grimms' tale of
"Fitcher's Bird" who held the key to the locked room where the remains of
many young maidens lay in bloody disarray. We must open the door to the
cell, wherein the Self and its love of authentic beauty were banished, and
see what carnage lies behind it.

The Evil That Lurks

Investing the lion's share of our ego in our public image comes with a hefty
price tag, far beyond the cost of our cosmetics and clothing. For when
women were separated from the ancient knowledge that our bodies are
the temples of spirit and that the true purpose of adornment is Self-
expression and praise, we were also severed from the truth about the
nature of our self-worth.

That's because the split from our Self negated the ancient knowledge
that we are worthy simply because we are part of Creation—simply
because we *are*. Instead, our stepsister ego sides with our culture's erroneous belief that we have no worth of our own, and that we must *create* it
via our appearance.

But having to compete publicly for self-esteem, places our ego on a
teeter-totter. If we feel good only when we mirror society's standards, we
inevitably plummet. Down goes the see-saw as soon as our latest look fades
from fashion, someone else buys better jewelry than ours, or we begin to
age despite our most recent surgery. So off we go to Bloomingdale's or the
plastic surgeon, and our ego rides high a little longer.

So why do we ride the teeter-totter that will ultimately let us down?
Because we who rely on a socially dictated appearance to give us a positive
sense of self find that there doesn't seem to be much of a self there when

we don't look "right." It seems that our only choice is to stay on the see-saw and strive for the highs.

But riding the teeter-totter can't give us the self-worth we so desperately seek, especially as we move into our middle decades, when our self-worth hinges on being firmly rooted in the Self. Unfortunately, in the long run we lose much more than we gain. And as illogical as it sounds, the loss may be even greater for those women who stay up the longest because of their natural physical beauty and the financial resources to buy the best age-reducing products. For when they finally fade, as they inevitably will, nothing can give them back the ego highs they once had, no matter how hard they try.

Does this mean that the rest of us, the women who never had perfect hair or an unlimited balance on their Saks credit cards, are outside the snare of the complex? Absolutely not. *All* women's self-worth, not just the attractive ones, hinge on society's stringent standards. Women who feel that they didn't, don't, couldn't, or can't physically measure up often suffer just as greatly.

I'm reminded of being introduced to a woman at my husband's tennis club who was friendly until a mutual acquaintance told her about me writing this book. Then she shut down like a cellar door before a storm. Turning away, she snapped out something about being an athlete who wasn't interested in beauty. I was embarrassed by her rudeness, but mainly I felt the excruciating pain that each of us carries in the name of parlor beauty.

Some women who've felt the sting of the narrow appearance standard pull in during their teens, never pushing past what they believe their lack of attractiveness limits them to and then failing to develop to their fullest. To make matters worse, on looking back in later years, they often realize their mistake but feel it's too late to make amends. Others, like the woman at the tennis club, turn bitter and cut off contact with or ridicule women they see as being more attractive, thereby robbing themselves of a wider circle of friends.

Alternatively, some women are like my friend Nancy's sister, Linda. Nancy, an attractive woman in her early forties, idly mentioned one day to Linda that as she ages, she misses men turning their heads as she enters restaurants and truck drivers whistling when she walks down the street. Whereupon Linda, the less attractive of the two, broke down in tears, because she'd never experienced that heady feeling of being admired for her beauty. Now that she's getting older, she mourns that she'll never know how it feels to have been beautiful.

Nancy and Linda's story clearly depicts the divergent and tragic nature of our situation. All of us—the born beautiful and those who fall somewhere outside society's rigid standards—are in the same leaky boat.

Self-Alienation

In *Women Who Run With the Wolves*, Clarissa Pinkola Estés tells how the goddesses of old brushed the hair of the women they loved most. What a glorious experience! Can't you picture elder high priestesses standing by the fire under a full moon lovingly washing and painting women's bodies during their rites of passage?

We, however, do not have permission to comb and stroke our sisters freely and openly. In fact, many of us recoil if we so much as brush up against another woman in the grocery line because the cut that severed us from our Self and focuses our attention on our appearance left us alienated from the very bodies we value so. Too, along with this love/hate relationship western society fostered on our bodies, its irrational and excessive fear of homosexuality squelched the primal joy that comes when women touch each other.

Nonwestern societies have taken for granted the small percentage of the population that prefers their own gender sexually. Yet they understand well that our desire to be touched, brushed, washed, clothed, and even fed by other women isn't sexual—sensual, yes; but not sexual.

I had a series of best friends in grade school, first Linda, then Marilyn, then Diane. We held hands and walked everywhere. We sat as close as we could, laughing till our heads fell on each other's shoulder. But innocent hand holding stopped in junior high, lest we be called "fruits." In high school we touched only in cumbersome hugs of comfort over broken relationships.

To quell our deeply buried need to be touched, women steal moments from hairdressers, masseuses, animals, and small children. Some of us even allow the occasional, sterile patty-pat of a close friend, but few would walk down the street holding hands with another woman, stroke her hair, or embrace her warmly for more than a split second.

Despite our phobias, however, we need to touch and be touched by other women as unabashedly as we did in girlhood. Touching deepens our connection with the feminine and sustains our love for our femaleness and female bodies the same as a mother's touch succors her growing child. This is especially true as our bodies age. We need physical reminders that our aging bodies are good and lovable, irrespective of their wrinkles and lumps.

Such pleasurable touching is verboten, however, not only because of the societal cringe that ensues, but because of the sexual baggage we carry. And do we ever carry the bags dumped on Eve's doorstep! We learned early on that our bodies weren't ours to enjoy for our own pleasure. Worse, men's assumed masterhood over our bodies opened the door for sexual invasion. In addition to the physical abuse some of us have suffered, we've all endured pornography, jokes about our sexuality, off-handed sexual innuendoes, sexual harassment at our jobs, and irreverent references to the shape, size, and color of our bodies.

Because of such invasion, we're literally "out of touch" with our bodies. Since we're cut off from the knowledge that they are ours and are innately good, the idea of touching ourselves for self-satisfaction has been a nonissue. In fact, I'd be willing to wager that most of us have never stroked our bodies out of love as we would pat children and animals. Contrarily, perchance we absentmindedly rub ourselves, we stop short— shamed by our own hand.

When it comes to our sexual body, we not only don't touch, we don't even look. A hilarious scene in the movie *Fried Green Tomatoes* finds middle-aged Evelyn fleeing a women's support group rather than pulling down her britches and looking at the reflection of her vagina in a hand mirror. Her plight is so funny because we can all relate to it. We weren't allowed to explore "down there" as children, and we're not about to at forty or fifty.

As I watched the film I remembered back to my mid-twenties when a psychologist friend told me that a woman couldn't be satisfied by some-one else unless she could satisfy herself. I was aghast. Good Texas girls didn't masturbate! We didn't even admit to knowing what the word meant. Many years and a lot of learning later I realized that his wisdom was centuries old.

On a less funny note, the scene from *Fried Green Tomatoes* probably caused theater audiences to giggle in shame at the very idea of a middle-aged woman *thinking* about her vagina, much less taking a peek at it. For when patriarchy damned menopausal women, they damned their sex-uality as well, and the older body was consigned to perpetual chastity. Only witches, who supposedly copulated with the devil himself, were thought to have had sex.

Attitudes haven't changed much. I wasn't too surprised at what one of my graduate students found when he analyzed the way women are depicted in advertisements in *Modern Maturity,* the mouthpiece for millions of older people. Despite a carefully crafted editorial policy that bars writ-ten material negatively slanted toward aging, a close assessment of a year's worth of advertisements revealed a powerfully negative visual statement.

Each ad for products such as vitamins and life insurance featured models in their fifties if not well past. Yet every model in ads for appearance-related products such as clothing and cosmetics was *at least* twenty years younger than those in the other ads. This nonverbal message about when older women are okay and when they aren't damages women, despite what Madison Avenue claims when criticized for how it portrays women.

For a fact, the message that only a young body is a worthy body *does* say that the aging body isn't sexually viable or alluring. The remake of the movie *Sabrina* brought the point squarely home for me. It wasn't only that Harrison Ford, my heart-throb since he cruised along Ventura Boulevard in *American Graffiti*, has now taken his place among middle-aged actors who fare best opposite young actresses. I thought of Audrey Hepburn, the consummate role model for my Sabrina years. Unlike many of her contemporaries, she matured into a model for how we might age in grace, talent, and natural beauty. But now she's been shoved aside by a younger Sabrina.

To be sure, constant reference in the media to the older woman's lack of acceptable sexuality trips us back into the Catch-22 of the narcissus complex. When we're shown over and again that only young flesh is desirable flesh, hundreds of thousands of us flee to the junior dress departments at our favorite stores.

Unrealized Potential

But being able to buy the same dress size that we wore in college isn't Self-affirming. It's just the opposite.

A TV commercial aired several years ago, which offers an example of the message sent by midlife women who still buy trendy, junior styles. After eating a low-fat cereal and losing weight, a mother is able to wear her teenage daughter's "rubber dress." This message is common in ads—use our product and look like a maiden. But at a deeper level, the real message a rubber dress sends is that a woman who remains looking like a teenager hasn't *developed* past adolescence. Think about it. The symbolic meaning of a tight, short, latex dress is not competence, maturity, creativity, and stability. It implies immaturity, even flakiness.

In ancient times, menopause was celebrated by meaningful rites of passage, during which a woman would have removed the symbols of her earlier stage and donned the clothing of the upcoming one. Anthropologists tell us that rites are powerful tools for instructing us on how to move from one stage of our lives to the next, otherwise we have little notion of what we should be like once we enter the next phase. Without them we can even slip into a more infantile state and have greater trouble emerging from it.

Yet, for all intents and purposes, society has done away with rites of passage. Those few that remain, such as baptisms, bat mitzvahs, sweet sixteens, and weddings, focus on maidens. And while these occasions usually require new clothes, the clothing often has been stripped of sacred symbolism in favor of expensive designer labels and, all too often, one upmanship.

In the best of all possible worlds, we would still have meaningful, spirit-filled rites for each stage in our life cycle, including our middle passage. But unfortunately, we're pretty much left on our own. So in one more way, our stepsister ego, egged on by our internalized stepmother, sits in the parlor and encourages us to remain at the lowest rung of the developmental ladder—that of the rubber dress.

This isn't to imply that we ignore our midlife passage altogether, but the few celebrations we have don't move us toward individuation. In fact, they openly support our complex. Social critics say that the face-lift is the rite of passage for the boom generation, and the color of choice for our fortieth and fiftieth birthday parties is black—not in commemoration of our up-coming cronehood, but as the color of death.

The underlying meaning of black balloons is far from innocent, however. In *Meeting the Madwoman,* Linda Schierse Leonard describes those who refuse to give up their youthful image. "Bitterness and a personal, inner ugliness are the fate of many a 'darling doll' who remain idle, relying on youth, charm, and beauty, failing to develop their talents and to embody their *inner* beauty."

There are also women who remind me of Helen Reddy's song about Delta Dawn with her rose pinned on, ever looking for her youthful lover. Although not bitter, they too look and act like child-women, never grasping the fullness of their womanhood and reaping the harvest of their yeasty midlife selves.

Women like these die to their later years because they suffer from one of the major disabling symptoms of the narcissus complex—the inability to look forward. Somewhere along the way they turn around and pin their eyes on the past, thereby losing out on the future.

I'm convinced that our unwillingness to face the future is why oldies music has taken over the radio airwaves. To be sure, part of the midlife passage requires that we look back and assess our lives so that we can make adjustments and go on. And since music of the times mirrored so closely who we were during our teens and twenties, listening to it is like entering a time machine so we can reflect back. Returning to the styles of our teens and twenties feeds our nostalgia for the same reason. But when I walk through the women's department at Nordstrom and see exact copies of Mary Quant mini-dresses from the 1960s or have friends who listen to nothing but the same old songs year in and year out, I quake in my boots. It seems that too many of us would rather collude with the stepmother and stay in a time warp than grow.

Fractured Trinity

Not only are we severed from the natural growth of our second half, but our insistence on maintaining our youth separates maidens, matrons, and crones from one another. That's because at the heart of the complex lies another deadly trait that Jung identified as commonplace among the unindividuated—jealousy.

Because we believe that an aging appearance means that we're past our prime, jealousy of the young runs rampant in this society. And the competition that jealousy creates in the family, the workplace, and society in general, causes untold misery, mistrust, and missed opportunities at every stage of our life cycle.

We could easily say that what Cinderella's stepmother does to her is mild when compared to the jealousy-driven evil done to most fairy tale maidens by older women. Snow White's stepmother couldn't find room in her heart to love herself, much less the maiden in her care. She turned yellow and green with rage when the mirror said that Snow White was the fairest in the land. Similarly, the old witch who turned beautiful maidens into nightingales in the tale of "Jorinda and Joringea" was yellow-colored.

Interestingly, green and yellow symbolize two of the most necessary ingredients of the individuation process—green means openness to growth and change, while yellow suggests integration. But even colors have their shadow sides. When associated with the Dark Mother, green and yellow become the colors of the unindividuated woman, the one who sees only the beauty of the young as the prize she craves for herself.

Snow White's stepmother hired a huntsman to kill the child and bring the girl's heart to her. But the hunter spared the child, killed a deer instead, and gave its heart to the stepmother, whereupon the evil queen ate it. By ingesting another's heart, one is believed to take on the other's positive characteristics, in this case, beauty. So in striving to maintain her appearance, the queen acted out the aspect of the Dark Mother that humankind fears most: The devourer.

This is nasty stuff! Yet, when western society split the Great Crone and projected only her dark side onto mature women, women were programmed to become devourers. For as I said earlier, the split-off, unintegrated, and unindividuated side of our natures degenerates into the stepmother who consumes us by disallowing our middle passage and the rich life it should bring. Then, in jealousy and frustration, we consume young maidens. For example, middle-aged women executives are notorious for blocking the career paths of younger women. And social dowager queens often place unnecessary and punitive demands on young women who wish to climb the social ladder.

Then too, when society measures female worth in youthful beauty, the possibilities for girl children maturing to their full potential is limited if not killed off altogether. The only thing Cinderella's mother asked as she lay dying was that her child remain good and pious—in other words to be true to and honor her Self. And when we birth a daughter, something deep in us asks the same for her. But when from birth on society chips away at everything that's not related to her appearance, it eats up her good and pious Self.

Too often society's desire for attractive little girls translates directly into mothers who live their own lives through their beautiful daughters, à la Cinderella's stepmother, who positions her daughters in the parlor. The stage mom is a classic example. But there are also thousands of less publicized mothers who live and die emotionally through their daughters, grooming and pushing them to be cheerleaders, prom queens, and beauty contestants.

The mother in Houston several years ago who plotted to kill the mother of her daughter's rival for a spot on the cheerleading squad sent waves of laughter through those circles who hadn't witnessed the deep-seeded need too many mothers have to see their daughters on the beauty ramp or the playing-field sidelines. The incident recalled to my mind a middle-aged woman I met at a workshop. The poor woman cried as though her heart would break for nearly a half hour because she still felt the anguish of failing to make her mother proud of her when she didn't win her hometown's Junior Miss pageant.

At first glance, we might want to blow off her reaction as a minor incident that happened over thirty years ago to a woman who is overly sensitive and underdeveloped. But her response to an event that should have merely been part of her adolescent growth is just the point I make. The hurt feelings in regard to parlor beauty that daughters receive from mothers are then passed on to their daughters, locking us all into a state of perpetual adolescence.

Then we have the mom who may not push her daughter into beauty-related enterprises, but who directly competes with her attractiveness—the rubber dress syndrome. Surely we don't believe that Demeter would have been better off merrily going out with Persephone to pick flowers. Persephone and Demeter weren't peers; they were two women in two special arcs of their life cycles, with specific responsibilities and distinct goals. But if Demeter tries to compete with Persephone's loveliness, the entire relationship changes, weakening if not negating altogether her mature nurturance, teaching, and guiding.

For generations, young people have demonstrated coming-of-age with looks that set them apart from their parents' generation. Our uncontrolled hair and tie-dyed T-shirts were the bane of our parents, just as our mothers' turned down hose and scruffy saddle oxfords bedeviled theirs. Up until recently, however, the young were left to their weird getups. But that's no longer the case. When I see my college sophomores and their moms both sporting Doc Martens™ I wonder who's raising whom.

Persephone didn't need another girlfriend in a rubber dress—and neither do our daughters. She needed a mature mother who could get her out of a jam by using all of her power, intuition, and wiles. Modern-day Persephones need mothers who are more like my friend Sarah. Shortly after she and her daughter, Michelle, had discussed what type of robe Michelle would need for her freshman year at college, Sarah had the following dream:

I come out of a dormitory wearing my favorite robe during my college years. But as I stepped onto the sidewalk, I felt that I wasn't dressed properly. So I went back into the dorm and put on the style of clothes I wear now.

This dream snippet powerfully symbolizes Sarah's wisdom concerning her daughter's upcoming transition into womanhood, her role in Michelle's transition, and her own midlife role. In the dream, it's Sarah, not Michelle, who's living in a dorm; yet when Sarah comes out wearing her own college robe, it doesn't feel right. She knows that Michelle, not she, belongs there. So Sarah goes back and changes out of her college robe (role) and into clothes that befit her current age and stage.

Sarah's dream clearly depicts the cord that binds maidens and matrons. Watching young women repeat the paths we took at their age reminds us of our earlier looks and roles. Seeing them brings up the ambiguity we feel as they do the wonderful things that young girls are supposed to do. But the difference between Sarah and those who are caught in the narcissus complex is that she deals with her feelings as a mature matron, one who views herself as having, if you will, "been there, done that" (albeit with some nostalgia). Clearly, Sarah feels comfortable and secure both in her midlife role and with her appearance.

It isn't just mothers and daughters who are separated from one another, women of all ages are. For lamentably, the looking glass comes between not only modern-day Demeters and Persephones but between Hecate and just about everyone. Because of society's ideas about who constitutes worth, our fear of death, and the vaulted position of the very young, modern maidens are too often unaware of the treasure that older women hold for them. This creates an arrogance that can result in a general disdain for any woman older than thirty-five. And because we in our mid-years also reflect society's contempt for all but the very young, we, too, turn our backs on our grandmothers as we look to our daughters for inspiration and truth.

Instead of honoring older women as gnarled and grayed high-priestesses, society sets them apart. Those who don't conform to ever playing the role of the maiden are shunned from the workplace and the social arena, so they don't offend our sense of beauty. This leaves our daughters cut off from the crone-wisdom they need in their time of budding, and we're denied that same wisdom during our midlife transition. Our crones suffer, too, for they're severed from the life's blood that nurturing maidens and matrons brings—roles they were programmed to perform thousands of years ago. It's no wonder that some turn bitter, feel useless, or develop chronic illnesses.

So, although society's insistence that we ever look the part of a teenager may seem harmless, it's not. The rubber-dress syndrome forces us to play out the role of wicked stepmother to ourselves, our daughters, our mothers, and our grandmothers. And unless we take positive steps to rewrite the script, we'll continue to act out the part of the Dark Mother as we move into our second half.

My Role Models

Take a few minutes and bring to mind images of the important little girls and women whom you remember in storybooks, movies, TV, and magazines of your childhood. Then go back and reflect on each character. By analyzing them in this way, you'll get a good idea of the impact socially idealized role models had on your developing self-image as well as how they helped to lay the foundation for your current parlor image.

You'll likely find on examination that each role model was a perfected image of society's standards of the beautiful child-woman and was known for her physical attractiveness above any other personal quality. To check this out, ask yourself what you can recall about each one. You'll probably conclude that the message you received is: *Base your ideal self on an attractive, young appearance, use your wits or talents only in conjunction with your appearance or if your appearance fails you, and change your appearance as necessary to keep up with society's standards.*

Your list may include young heroines who were not known for their beauty, such as Anne of *Anne of Green Gables*. But even she wasn't without a measure of parlor-ego—Anne despised her red hair and accidentally dyed it green while trying to get rid of it!

As your list progresses from maidens to matrons, it may dwindle down to a paltry few entries. In its brevity and lack of women of real substance, wisdom, and power, however, a short list makes a strong point. For the greater part, the physical image that adult women impart via the media is either one of dowdiness (the good mothers) or of overdrawn, cartoonish flamboyance (the comediennes and buffoons). The only physically attractive and powerful middle-aged women are the devouring mothers. There are plenty of examples of such celluloid mothers-from-hell, from Joan Crawford's Mildred Pierce to *The Graduate's* Mrs. Robinson.

You can probably also recall many images of evil crones, such as the Wicked Witch of the West or Bette Davis' hideous character in *Hush, Hush Sweet Charlotte*. Regardless of who she was, however, the childhood images you received of the death-related crone seeped deeply into your unconscious only to rear its head as you now see your body take on the dreaded look of the older woman.

The few exceptions to the old-is-evil image probably didn't place the older woman in much better light. Although Granny Clampett wasn't evil, she hardly inspired confidence in the aging process or made you want to get there. And the few older women who were viable, fun, and confident, such as Auntie Mame, were portrayed as being somewhere left of center—part of the lunatic fringe that claims those women who won't age quietly. But in fact, Mame's appearance was authentic from her hat to her shoes. So look around again, there *are* good role models in the media, you just have to readjust your sights so you can recognize them.

➤ Four

Fatherless:
The Lure of the Label

After Cinderella's stepsisters took her pretty clothes and banished her to the kitchen, they mocked her and said, "Just look at the proud princess, how dressed up she is!"

When you read this story as a child, did you ever wonder why Cinderella's father didn't step in and help her? Surely her nightly absence from the parlor clues him in that something has happened to her. But he never acknowledges her plight. It's as though he forgets about her once the good mother dies. And in fact, that's precisely what happens. Once his first wife dies, the father soon abandons their child.

Just as Cinderella wasn't alone among fairy tale maidens in being motherless, she's one of hundreds who are fatherless. Although the fathers usually don't die, they tend to either abdicate their responsibilities to their daughters after the first wife dies, as do Cinderella's and Snow White's, or sell them out in some way as did Rapunzel's, the handless maiden's, and Sleeping Beauty's. Either way, they leave the maidens in want of fatherly protection.

To answer the question of why these fathers treat their daughters so poorly, we must remember that just as with the fairy tale mother, the father is an archetype, representing the highest ideal of the masculine character. As such, mythological fathers and kings symbolize the enabler, the doer, the one who sets the pace for how to live. They stand for power, order, discipline, and loyalty, as well as mastery and accomplishment.

It's well to remember that when we analyze the masculine archetype, it doesn't pertain just to men and how they think and act. All of us, women as well as men, have a masculine element—just as everyone has a female side. So when I discuss the fairy tale father as representing an archetype, I'm talking about the masculine principle within each individual as well as the masculine aspect of our society.

In prepatriarchal stories, the male ruler's might was balanced through marriage to a queen or devotion to a goddess whose love, nurturance, and belief in human equality tempered his power and assertiveness. Thus he ruled his kingdom, be it a country or his home, wisely, fairly, and with a loving hand.

Before she dies, Cinderella's mother could have balanced the father in this way, then he could have cared for his family with love and compassion. But after the good mother's death, everything changes. The story parallels what happened when patriarchy split the feminine. The father buries the loving wife and marries the soulless stepmother, and this marriage leaves him wounded for lack of the complete, balancing feminine. So he becomes as soulless as his new wife.

You can't just bury something as necessary as love, however. Inasmuch as the only thing we know about the father is that he's wealthy, we know how he fills the void. He substitutes love for money. Yet it isn't just money that the loveless father craves. Jung maintained that the opposite of love isn't hate, but power. So in his wounded condition, the father craves the kind of *power* that money buys. In his new way of thinking after his good wife's death, he like our society believes that possessions bestow the power he craves. And the more he has, the more esteem he gets from others.

The Possessing Father

Now that we understand what the father represents, we can better answer the question as to why he fails to protect Cinderella. As a man in medieval times, he prized owning fashionably attired maidens, for they bespeak of his high position in society. For although the stepsisters' life in the parlor may seem all sunshine and roses, make no mistake, they're there only to please the father's vanity with their commodity-based beauty. And since Cinderella is the child who knows the truth about spirit-based beauty, she has no place in either his heart or home. So he gladly steps aside when the stepsisters banish her to the kitchen.

Similarly, real fathers in our society abandon the Cinderella in their little girls—that part of us who retains the Mother's knowledge of our authenticity and unique worth. Even though modern fathers may believe that they raise their daughters with unconditional love, they're predisposed to control them—mold them to reflect their own needs, personalities, beliefs, and behaviors, as well as use them to display their wealth. For remember, since the death of the Great Mother, generations of fathers have been wounded. Like Cinderella's father, real-life fathers also force out everything in their daughters that bespeaks of the true mother.

Because our father abandons our Cinderella, by age two or three, most of us also abandon her. After all, we want more than anything in the world to be the apple of our dad's eye: And if earning his love means chasing that free-spirited little girl into the kitchen, so be it. We curb our tongues, bodies, ideas, and spontaneity in deference to being pretty to get daddy's attention. For being loved for half of who we are beats not being loved at all.

This dynamic rings true for both little girls who meet the approval of their father's eye and those who don't. Elaine had her father's full attention until she was three years old, when her sister, Susan, was born. Susan's fair hair and big blue eyes stole their father's heart, and she became his Susie-Q. Elaine, who'd inherited her mother's dark, stocky eastern European genes, sided with her mother. Although each sister's relationship with their father differed vastly, they both learned the same lesson— that the little girl who looks like she belongs in daddy's parlor fares better with him.

It wouldn't have occurred to Elaine and Susan's dad that anything in his household was amiss, however. Cinderella's tale tells us why. Given that Cinderella's father believed that he owns his daughters, he would also assume that they *should* look as he likes. If a daughter looked or dressed differently, then she was bad and subject to abandonment. For in his house, he presides as judge and jury.

This explains why modern-day men so often try to control how we look. Most of us can easily recall times when our fathers, brothers, husbands, lovers, or bosses let us know in no uncertain terms how we were *supposed* to look. In fact, it's so common that many of us don't even question their authority over our appearance. We're programmed to wear high heels at our husband's request even though our back aches at night or refrain from buying that red dress because *he* doesn't like the color.

I'm reminded of the time in high school when my father took away my car until I quit back-combing my hair so much. He had a valid point in that my hair *did* look like a rat's nest. But his reaction was far more than a mere difference in taste. Just as some mothers try to link themselves to their daughters' youth by wearing teenage styles, fathers often try to control their daughters' femininity and budding sexuality by controlling their appearance.

Shame

Little girls who violate the parlor rules about how they should look are humiliated unmercifully, just as was Cinderella. Even if looking right wasn't a mandate in our own households, society took up the slack—teachers, playmates, and relatives often play the father's role of shaming us into looking a certain way. Before long, our egos learn to play the father internally so that we shame ourselves relentlessly if we don't measure up to society's standards. So as we stand at the gates of middle age, we chide ourselves silently about baggy knees and thickening waists.

Unfortunately, we don't confine this shaming to ourselves. Those who have been destroyed know only to destroy others, so we who've been shamed learn early on how to ridicule how other women look. Thus we reap another whammy from the narcissus complex, for inasmuch as our desire for youthful beauty separates us from our mothers and daughters, the shaming we receive divides us from our sisters.

Like the stepsisters who mock Cinderella's appearance long after they banish her, we who've earned the prized seat next to the parlor fire don't simply rest in our good fortune. Since the looks that earn us the love we so desperately need are defined for us, we feel perfectly justified in shaming those sisters who don't conform to them.

We were trained at our father's knee (be it the wounded masculine archetype in our dads, our moms, or society) to judge others harshly—to believe that *we* are good and right and *they* are bad and wrong. That's why we ridicule the heavyset woman behind her back or snipe about someone's outfit as soon as she leaves the room.

By cutting down another woman's appearance, we momentarily alleviate the hurt of having been shamed when we failed to live up to other's *shoulds* regarding our own appearance. We try to shift the load of pain—maybe if we pass it on to some other woman, our wounds will heal. But, of course, they don't. Ridiculing others to relieve our ache over being severed from our Cinderella and then shamed if she dared raise her head is akin to rubbing salt into all the old cuts we've received along the way. It only makes them refester.

Since friends know that I study women's relationship to appearance, they sometimes ask me why someone looks the way she does: "Why would so-and-so want to look like that? Just who's she trying to impress?" Actually, I don't know why someone looks the way she does, unless I know her really well. Even then, I'm not sure and wouldn't say so if I did. But the question lets me know what the questioner thinks about *her* appearance. Jung called this transference of self-disdain *projection*. For when we're critical of other women's appearance, it's a sure indication that our internal father/judge is critical of us.

But try as we may to project our hurts onto others, they only come mirroring back to us. For when we slice another woman's appearance because she's young and reminds us of what we miss, is dressed in a way we can't afford, or looks like she belongs to a political, ethnic, social, or economic group different from ours, we merely lay raw our *own* feelings of shame.

Father Power

Like Cinderella's father, our culture believes that the more people own, the more respect and love they will garner. Money equates to social power because it secures one's position—allowing an individual or a nation to defeat the weak, conquer those higher up, and fend off one's position from those below. It's not too surprising then that the ladder to success is studded with status symbols, for they remind us of just who is who.

Patriarchy didn't invent status symbols. Since superior personal strength, wit, and talent helped earliest humans to survive, the most able, whether at hunting or healing, were rewarded with feathers, gold, fur, or whatever object the clan held sacred. But the difference between modern-day symbols and earlier ones is that early status symbols were earned by those who contributed to the good of the community, and they retained their holy meanings when worn.

In Old Europe midwives wore owl feathers to symbolize their link to the crone goddess and her power. Given human nature, I'm sure the midwives were personally pleased to wear the feathers. But the feathers didn't laud them as being better than women who weren't midwives and, therefore, unqualified to wear the sacred owl symbol.

But that changed. As women were stripped of their primal stature and forced to sit in the father's parlor as symbols of *his* position, we learned that a status-clad appearance is one of our only means of wielding power—of getting what we want, controlling others, and positioning ourselves in society. And while women of all ages wear economically-based status symbols, older women are especially prone to donning them to boost their sense of self-worth as the body ages. For without other socially-acceptable means, how else can they maintain a sense of personal value?

So, gemstones worn by our foremothers because they pulsated with nature's energy and reflected the colors of the deities now conspicuously display wealth. Rather than sing of sun and moon, gold and silver now rank a woman's social position. Animal skins no longer declare the oneness of life, but scream of vanity-based slaughter. In recent decades, designer logos came onboard along with the polished look of those who can afford the best skin, body, and hair care.

Status symbols are valuable because they are scarce. If they weren't, we could all afford them, and they couldn't indicate rank. What this boils down to, is that only a few sisters can sit in the parlor, and among those who do, the women with the most, best, and newest sit closest to the fireplace. And when it comes to the fight against aging, we can add those with the most to spend on reconstructive surgery and expensive antiaging products.

When we measure power in carats, however, we can't help but regard those who have the most as the worthiest and those who come up short as insignificant. So instead of viewing other women as equals and allies, as in the days of old, we compete with them. On seeing another woman, before we can blink, we run down a comparative checklist: size, age, beauty, cost. Then we judge her on each point. How much more? How much less?

Not even microwaves move information faster through some circles of women than news of someone getting a new ring. Shortly after a friend, who is my age, bought a diamond solitaire, I accidentally overheard two older women just as one relayed the information to the other; whereupon the second woman retorted in a matter-of-fact tone, "Mine's bigger." Obviously this woman was threatened. Like Snow White's stepmother, she turned green and yellow with envy and ran to the mirror to check to see if she was still the fairest in the land.

It's the old see-saw ride again. Because we've been convinced that our power hinges on our appearance, we look at other women and think, "If she's got more, I must be less." Or we gladly affirm, "If she's got less, I must be higher. If I'm higher, I must be better."

But is this genuine power? Of course not. In fact, it's just the opposite.

On reflection, we who are enamored by the father's power often find that the first part of our lives seems to have been lived in a fog—distant and unconnected. That's because when we devalue our authentic Selves while children and compensate for the loss of our genuine power by competing with other people for status and appearance-based worth, we *are* separated—both from our Selves and from them. As a child, I often perceived myself as living behind a plateglass window and everyone else as living on the other side of it. When I began my inner work, I had visions of myself as a child putting my nose up to the glass pane and enviously watching other children play, much as one would put her nose up to a store window and look at the out-of-reach Christmas toys on the other side.

As we grow up feeling separated, we learn to substitute this inferior, I-am-here-and-you-are-there feeling for one that says, "I am protected from you by my superior appearance or my thinness or my lack of wrinkles. As such, I can control who comes near me, and I'm able to protect myself from further hurt with my ice-queen demeanor." It's no coincidence that the jewels we wear are called ice and rocks, and we wrap ourselves in furs—clothing of those who live on barren, frozen land—thus symbolically freezing out other people while trying to warm up our chilly bones.

On the surface it may seem that owning the best connotes the might that gives us back some of the esteem we feel we lose as we age. In this we may believe that we're playing a zero/sum-based game in which the winner takes all, but instead the wounded father's contest ends up in a lose/lose situation for everyone.

King Fashion

Wait a minute, you might say. Women's bodies are no longer owned by men as they were in the Middle Ages. And of course that's true—but women are still dominated by a wounded-masculine principle that rivals any fairy tale father—the fashion industry. Seventh Avenue sets the standards for who sits in the parlor, and to understand just how much control fashion wields over us, let's take a look at a story whose main character has the all-time worst appearance-related narcissus complex in history—the emperor in Hans Christian Andersen's "The Emperor's New Clothes."

A vain emperor was approached by two swindlers who claimed they could make clothes that were invisible to everyone who wasn't fit for office. The emperor eagerly agreed to give the swindlers the gold they asked for; and they set to work making the invisible cloth. Various officials, and finally the emperor himself, came to see the fabric. But, of course, they couldn't see anything. Rather than letting on, however, each declared what fine cloth the tailors were making. Finally the day came when the emperor pretended to put on the new clothes and paraded through the city. The people cheered and exclaimed how beautiful the clothes were—all but a small child who told it like it was: The emperor wasn't wearing any clothes. With that, a cry went up in the streets that the emperor didn't have any clothes on.

Although a shiver went down the emperor's spine when he heard the jeers, he couldn't admit the truth. So, he and his entourage raised their heads higher and paraded on. And the swindlers rode out of town with the emperor's money.

In the story the emperor's desire for social power and the esteem it brings causes him to be targeted by tricksters. Tricksters surface in stories to balance conditions that have become too one-sided, turning everything topsy-turvy by poking fun at the mighty and the proud and creating the chaos out of which change comes. Too, they provide comic relief when our lessons become too hard to handle.

Who better to trick the vain emperor than a couple of swindlers making themselves out to be tailors? Mercury was the patron planet of medieval tailors, and Mercurius was the trickster god. And how better to trick the emperor than by selling him clothing that's invisible to all but those who are fit for office? These tricksters propose the ultimate in fashion—a fail-safe way to separate the worthy from the unworthy.

Tricksters may provide comic relief in stories, but the real-life swindler is far from funny. When society set the mechanics in motion whereby it ranks women according to how well we conform to a standardized look, it unwittingly licensed Seventh Avenue—the fashion industry—to render invisible those who are too unfashionable, overweight, poor, ignorant, or obviously too old to sit with the rest of us.

As much as we might not want to admit it, some women's lack of fashionable visibility causes others to ignore them as though they aren't even there. I call the expression we wear when we spy someone who doesn't measure up the "charity auction stare." It's my pet name for women's nonresponse to the less parlor-worthy that I first became aware of as a child when I watched a fellow worshipper at church. She was fascinating—blond, dressed to the nines—and she had a distant look in her eyes as she scanned the crowd for those with whom she cared to chat. Although at age ten I thought this woman's demeanor was cool, years later it troubled me—having seen it too often, having done it too often myself, and having come to understand it as nothing more than a defense against losing the parlor game.

In contrast to our unfashionably invisible sisters, society assigns the highest worth to women who visibly measure up. Magazines like *People* even tell us who counts nationally via best-dressed and most beautiful lists. From Manhattan to Muskogee, the visibly worthy show up in the society pages and sit atop A-lists.

I was amused by a well-known West Coast fashion-trend analyst who told me that by the end of the twentieth century individuality in dress would be the central fashion focus. He waived a photograph of Barbra Streisand as the upcoming model for older women. But when I asked him if individuality in older women of all sizes, incomes, heritages, and ethnicities would be welcomed equally on the covers of *Vanity Fair*, he smugly gave me a charity auction stare.

Stripping the Goddess

Though it caters to women customers, today's fashion industry is every bit a wounded-masculine enterprise. Once sacred to the Goddess herself, cloth now comes from high-tech looms where shuttles are thrust in greed rather than praise. Their hollow banging sings not of the holy but clatters of the competition, power, and control that their products symbolize.

Yet this isn't what we're told by the wizards of fashion. Like the emperor at the hands of the swindlers, we're led to believe that what comes from Seventh Avenue's looms is beautiful, creative, and mysterious. But as Kathleen Norris says in *Parabola* magazine, "Fashion designers are always trivial—that's what makes their pronouncements on the deeper meaning of the clothes so deliciously ludicrous."

Our clothes no longer have deep meaning because they're bereft of warmth, creativity, and individuality; in fact, mass produced fashions are so similar they could be designed by a single person. The same impersonalization can be said for our cosmetics. They're made of who-knows-what and cruelly tested on animals, then we buy them from mannequin-perfect women in lab coats. And they're so well-packaged and protected behind glass that we don't dare ask to examine them before we take them home.

At this point in our disconnection from appearance as Self-reflection, many of us don't even choose the *colors* we wear. Color analysts, who have no regard for which hues ring in harmony with our spirits, coolly look at our skin tones and send us off with prepared packets of swatches that we dutifully match. Similarly, we turn to wardrobe consultants to tell us what to buy and fashion magazine editors to tell us fashion do's and don'ts based on national trends. We diet and rely on plastic surgeons to make us conform to a single, youthful standard, regardless of our genes.

Over the past decades, a group of women have emerged in society who might at first glance seem impervious to the old system. We who are referred to as fathers' daughters stepped off of the traditional female path and followed our dads into the boardroom, operating room, and laboratory. But old ways hold fast, and our transformation didn't include giving up the fashion treadmill. We merely traded the parlor for the judges' chamber and our grandmother's tea gown and pearls for Brooks Brothers™ suits and Rolex™ watches. Indeed, boom generation women rank among the most status-conscious in history.

To keep the millions of us who went directly from college to corporation on course, the fashion industry created a new concept: *power* dressing. A couple of years ago when a Reebok ad showed sweaty women working out, power walking, and mountain biking along with such captions as, "I believe in taking the path less traveled," we might have felt some independence. But if we look closely, the ad *really* reads, "You are powerful *only* when you wear our prestigious brand." So what's new? This new-woman-of-the-'90s trick created a multimillion dollar payback for the industry and didn't liberate us one bit. We're still as afraid as ever that we're going to grow old and become invisible.

The Powers That Be

After the emperor gives the swindlers the gold they ask for, he becomes rife with curiosity about their progress and sends his lord high Chamberlain to look in on them. Although the emperor reassures himself that he is more than fit for his position, he nevertheless dispatches his most competent aide to check out the work first.

Our narcissus complex sees to it that we can never be too sure about ourselves either. Even as we stand on the threshold of our powerful Hecate decades, we have little basis for feeling lovable in and of ourselves. In fact, like the stepsisters who remain under the father's thumb, we tend to feel *more* at other people's mercy. Even a long look in the mirror to confirm that we look up to snuff isn't enough, because deep down we fear that we might not measure up even if we *seem* to appear okay.

To assuage our fear we turn to others to tell us that we look okay and, therefore, *are* okay. Each metropolis and burg has its fashion mavens, the ones who know how to dress and to whom others turn for advice, and nationally we rely on *Vogue*'s monthly advice. After all, aren't they, like the Chamberlain, the ones who can be trusted above all others?

Perhaps not. The Chamberlain refuses to acknowledge that he failed to see any fabric, causing the emperor eventually to parade before the whole city in his BVDs. Similarly, our ability to assume that the women on the local best-dressed list and those who put together the glossy magazines have our genuine interest at heart is equally tenuous.

Instead, too often the fashion mavens themselves are so caught up in the narcissus complex that they rule like dowager queens, complete with an entourage of well-dressed maidens and matrons. Yet these crones are no wise and caring Hecates. They sit next to the fireplace and wield their loveless power over younger women like stepmothers—making or breaking their charges, depending on how well they look the part and play the game. And beware, these *grand dames* will fling any young maiden who threatens their honored position into the bowels of the kitchen.

The tricksters knew darn well that the old Chamberlain wouldn't spill the beans. Similarly, the fashion industry knows that those who stake their reputations, worth, and social positions on them won't either. For in exposing the system, they would be forced to expose their dependency on it. Let's face it, if women weren't slaves to fashion and felt completely free to express their individuality, there would be no need for fashion dictators.

The glowing reports from the trusted Chamberlain entices the emperor to inspect the fabric personally, and he wends his way to the swindlers with his full entourage in tow. But as he looks into the empty looms, the awful truth stares back. Is he unfit to be emperor because he can't see the cloth? Absolutely not! He maintains his composure and exclaims, "It's wonderful, just wonderful." Whereupon the entourage proclaims the nonexistent fabric wonderful, too.

It's no different today. Year after year semiannual fashion collections are ushered in with lavish pomp on runways in Paris, Milan, and New York. And season in, season out, the styles are so hideous, unflattering, and contrived that no woman in her right mind would wear them. Be that as it may, the empresses of style—the international fashion editors— laud each collection. Then the courtiers—the retail buyers, fashion coordinators, fashion press, and best-dressed reply, "Indeed! Most Excellent! Marvelous!"

The New Pantheon

To make sure that no one suspects the truth, the emperor caps his praise of the wondrous fabric by proclaiming the swindlers "Knights of the Loom." Such acclaim is also commonplace in today's fashion industry.

Marie Antoinette's dressmaker, Rose Bertin, was the first fashion designer to be known by name. Prior to her, royal dressmakers were personal servants whose names were never recorded. Over the years, however, society elevated fashion designers from anonymous dressmakers to national icons. Not only do modern designers rub shoulders with their clients but more often than not are themselves the honored guests.

These days the visit of a famous designer to an up-scale store is akin to a royal appearance down to the last detail. The celebrity is preceded by advance people who come in to check out arrangements and apprise the store's staff of the designer's special sensitivities. The store's best patrons blatantly jockey for invitations to various events—with seating near the designer-celebrity a most serious matter. Above all hangs the ever-present threat of a temper tantrum by the Seventh Avenue guru should something be amiss. That not one of those whom I talked with about such visits would allow me to quote her, give the name of her store, or reveal her identity in any way, for fear of losing her job, attests to the power these latter-day deities hold.

Perfectionism

It was told that the emperor had a different robe for each hour of the day. He reminds me of a middle-aged woman I know, Caroline, who also has a massive wardrobe and spends a fortune on being the first to wear the latest style, owning the best jewelry, and sporting the most expensive furs.

Ironically however, Caroline rarely goes anywhere without phoning a friend to find out what *she's* wearing. This may seem a bit strange, given that Caroline's goal is to sit closest to the fireplace, but it really isn't. Caroline really doesn't call up friends to find out what they plan to wear so that she can copy it. Looking identical to her friends is the farthest thing from her mind. Although Caroline couldn't explain it in so many words, she calls to find out what *look* is appropriate. Then she bests it.

Caroline spends all this energy perfecting her appearance because deep down she's afraid not to. That's because women in the throes of the narcissus complex commonly feel a compulsion to be the ultimate. In *The*

Impostor Phenomenon, Pauline Rose Clance says, "For perfectionists, the thought of easing up and expecting less of themselves creates almost immediate panic. The reason for this fear is because of an underlying belief that they must be perfect in order to be lovable."

We see the wounded father's handprint in this. A woman like Caroline internalized the belief that other people dispense love the same as they give birthday presents. As a child she wanted so desperately to be daddy's pretty ballerina. Today, she still wants love from those around her, so she goes overboard on her appearance in order to get it.

Abandonment

The emperor was so obsessed with his appearance that he abdicated his other duties in favor of public outings that provided opportunities to display his vast wardrobe. Since many of us learned early on that what we do and say is much less important than how we look doing and saying it, we also abandon other responsibilities to the back of the closet. For example, Caroline stays very busy. Yet, if you watch carefully you realize that her focus really isn't on what she's doing at all. The focal point of her life is what she has on, what she has recently purchased to wear, and what she plans to wear in the future.

This is because we who are obsessed with our appearance cannot just let it go once we've dressed ourselves. How we look is too near and dear to our hearts to leave it on our makeup table and behind our closet door. Instead, we stay glued to our appearance wherever we go rather than contemplating issues, generating ideas, creating, or simply listening to and learning from others. Thus we see that we repeat the father's abandonment of Cinderella in our own lives. We let go of all but that which allows us to stay in the parlor.

Carried to an extreme, we get so caught up in the mirror as we age that we abandon far more than interests and ideas. When Caroline's son got involved with drugs, she sent him back east to a military school rather than deal with it. Since Caroline is so disconnected from her innate feminine, she simply didn't have the wherewithal to cope with her son's neediness. Then, over the next year, she upped the ante appearance-wise and invested in several pieces of expensive jewelry—an antidote many women use to alleviate the complex problems they face as they move into middle age.

If like Caroline we fail to attach deep meaning to anything except our appearance, by the time we reach our middle decades, we also have no means of tapping our inner resources when life makes its sudden turns. We're left with only one means of patching up the psychic energy that bleeds us dry when life's tragedies beset us; we cover the wounds with a perfected, packaged look.

In addition to being lame when it comes to reaching down and pulling up strength and know-how as we turn forty, fifty, or sixty, we who feel the pinch of perfectionism are further hamstrung as we age because we cannot cope with failure. As maidens we either never tried or quickly abandoned activities that required tenacity, for we were incapable of dealing with the failures inherent in making a successful relationship, career, or project. So now, when faced with the failures that inevitably precede success in our midlife ventures, we concentrate harder on creating an appearance that proves we are perfect without all the struggle. But beware, the call to turn inward is too strong and cannot be smothered in finery or smoothed away by surgeons.

The Public Eye

The emperor's all-time favorite pastime was parades. We who maintain our sense of worth via a power-based appearance also thrive on being out and being seen. And in an effort to avoid public invisibility as our youthful looks wane, remaining front and center via a well-crafted appearance can become an obsession. Caroline's social engagements are so much a part of her sense of self that she carries a date book stuffed full of invitations. Throughout the day she pulls it out and checks it—always in open view of whomever is around her. Others of us support our parlor ego with a Day-Timer™ filled with business meetings, lunches, and after-hours events.

When our sense of self floats atop a tide of social approval, we stay in constant view of everyone because being alone is frightening. For, when we are alone, no one is there to love us. So we avoid solitude at every cost, even if it means calling up a friend to come over and play cards on the only night we've had alone in the past six months.

The absence of solitude, however, again threatens us with a deadly complex-produced toxin as we move into our mid years. Although we who are trapped by the mirror stay the busiest, we're rarely the ones who do the best work, think the most enlightened thoughts, create the best art, or make the greatest strides. For in truth, accomplishment comes through the combination of dedication and solitude. As Anthony Storr writes in *Solitude,* "the capacity to be alone is necessary if the brain is to function at its best, and if the individual is to fulfill [her] highest potential. Human beings easily become alienated from their own deepest needs and feelings. Learning, thinking, innovation, and maintaining contact with one's own inner world are all facilitated by solitude." Thus when we fail to honor our need to be alone, the father's thumb extracts one more pound of our flesh and fosters a death on us not unlike Narcissus'.

Conformity

On the morning of the big procession, the emperor strips down to his skivvies and feigns delight as he pretends to don his costly, new wardrobe. With each piece, the courtiers gush out obligatory oooohs and aaaahs. Similarly, the good citizens cheer in wild approval as the emperor passes by.

Like those who laud the emperor even though he's all but naked, we all too often dress so we won't look different from everyone else. And this doesn't go just for those who wear elitist fashion, either. The hippies of the '60s and '70s mandated a counterculture look. Other groups eschew costly clothes for commonsense styles based on frugality. Still others bank on dressing for business success. And as I've pointed out so often, middle-aged women often feel that to remain viable, they must adhere to the styles in *Elle* and *Mademoiselle,* magazines geared to women in their late teens and twenties. So the issue isn't *what* we wear, it's the belief that we *must* wear a proscribed look to be welcome in our group's parlor. But most of us never stop to analyze how, why, or by whose authority *they* are what author Terry Lynn Taylor calls the cool police. We just assume that *they* are right and follow along.

As children we were expected to conform to our family's look. Anything more or less was shameful. In our teens we were further split from our Cinderella-like selves. But as Mary Pipher says in *Reviving Ophelia,* "This time the pressure comes not from parents but from the culture. Adolescence is when girls experience social pressure to put aside their authentic selves and to display only a small portion of their gifts." We learn to rank our peers from cool to nerdy, based on the brands of their clothing and the stores where they shop.

Sadly, however, what we learned as maidens doesn't evaporate over time. As young matrons we moved from high school to college, to job, to motherhood by handling difficult tasks with great aplomb, but we never got past believing that if we didn't fit in with how *they* look, then we were not as good as *they* were. Now that we are older and even more accomplished, despite our achievements, the fright about not being good enough continues to haunt us. This is sad, but it more than explains why the emperor's subjects feign wild approval of his invisible clothes.

The Naked Truth

The townspeople shout with approval, that is, until a child gasps, "But the emperor hasn't got any clothes on!" And then they jeer.

It would make sense that a child exposed the sham because children are innocent of do's and don'ts about what to wear when until they are contaminated by society. Then they demand clothes from Baby Gap™. Given free reign and a variety of choices, however, a child with her Cinderella intact dresses from her intuition and imagination, not from TV ads and sitcoms.

Too, until contaminated, children are honest. They see through fashion hoopla and laugh at an outrageous look at the drop of a designer hat. As children, my cousins and I spent many a summer afternoon mimicking the models' stiff poses and breaking up with laughter at the styles in *Harper's Bazaar*. But of course, as we moved from grade school to junior high that all changed—we closed our inner eyes and ears, and *Seventeen* became our Bible.

In the emperor's story, the courtesans, too, close their eyes to the truth. They surely know in their heart-of-hearts that they're parading in front of the whole town behind a near-naked emperor while pretending to hold up his nonexistent train. Yet they hold on. Their esteemed positions are linked to the emperor, so they can't afford to see the sham. And the emperor closes his ears. It isn't that he doesn't hear the crowd's jeers. We know he does—he gets goose bumps. But the truth can't penetrate because his heart is frozen. The emperor pays no more attention to the child's words than Cinderella's father heeds her whimpers as she weeps in the kitchen.

These men's hearts are frozen because the wounded masculine operates from an estranged ego. With no link to the Self, it runs on machismo. Do or die, he must be right; he must, as the advertising slogan warns, never let them see him sweat.

In the same way, our wounded society refuses to acknowledge the damage done to women when our social worth and personal power are measured in finery. It isn't that we haven't heard words of warning. The dirty little secret that the fashion system fails women big time is public knowledge. *The Beauty Myth* stayed on the bestseller list for months and was preceded and followed by at least half-a-dozen similar books.

But when the collective shiver is over, when the books slip from the lists, and the authors no longer are welcome guests on "Oprah," society holds its head higher, its charity auction stare a little longer, and continues on. The courtiers—the media, Madison Avenue, and the medical and pharmaceutical professions—hold on even tighter, clinching their fists in fear of what might happen if society heeds the orphan in the kitchen.

Those of us who stake our social worth on prescribed fashion also are reluctant to face the truth, even when presented with evidence that it has cost us dearly in the past and will rob us of the fullness of our upcoming decades. We don't want to be the first on our block to admit the lie because like the courtesans, we feel that we simply have too much to lose. So we hold on tight to what we have and parade on.

The Price Tag

We who hold on, however, are akin to the caterpillars in Trina Paulus' *Hope for the Flowers*. The caterpillars spend their lives climbing up on top of each other—clawing other's backs, pushing down the weak. Yet if and when they make it to the top, they don't find anything up there except the caterpillars who've also gotten there. There's no other reward.

For certain the climb doesn't make them better caterpillars. In fact, those who make it to the top are jaded by the struggle and disdain those whom they clawed on the way up. Some even fall off and are killed. And those who survive aren't that much better off. Their single-minded goal of reaching the top robs them of their natural birthright to turn inward, spin cocoons, and then live out their lives as beautiful, free butterflies.

So it is with us. We're reluctant to assess the actual price we pay to sit in the parlor as we age. For when we do, we discover that staying with the appearance chase is as virulent to our midlife individuation as is the caterpillars' climb. Instead of making us better, our dependence on our parlor image over our lifetime leaves us merely older and too often also hardened, cynical, and mean-spirited. For when the father joins up with his new wife and stepdaughters, he teaches them how to climb with the best. But he fails to tell them that there is no lasting reward for sitting pretty in his parlor—nothing covering the naked emperor, nothing at the top of the caterpillar mound, and nothing atop the fashion heap.

I'm not implying that wanting to look good and have beautiful clothing is wrong or will lead to self-destruction. As I've said over and again, these are *natural* desires. What's wrong is the system that co-opted our Cinderella knowledge about authentic appearance and replaced it with one-size-fits-all parlor clothes that are supposed to last us from cradle to grave.

Make no mistake, the clothes and shoes that were taken from Cinderella represent much more than a mere difference in style from that preferred by the stepsisters. As the child of the good mother, Cinderella would have learned to adorn herself authentically from the love in her heart and in praise of spirit. But the loveless father has absolutely no appreciation for what her clothes represent. All he knows is to put down her Self-inspired appearance. So there's no way our internal wounded-father and wicked stepmother are going to honor our midlife drive to turn away from the glitzy parlor, adorn ourselves in authenticity, and learn about our innate goodness and unique talents.

Who's Pulling Your Appearance Strings?

This quiz will tell you the extent you let other's "shoulds" control your appearance. Read each statement carefully, then respond with the word *always*, *often*, *sometimes*, or *never*.

- I feel that I should have something new and different to wear for special occasions (by special, I don't mean your wedding, I mean a friend's).
- I feel that other women look better than I.
- I ask my friends what they're wearing before I decide what to wear.
- I will not wear certain styles or colors because someone (mother, father, friend, lover, consultant) has said that they are (childish) (matronly) (not my style) (unflattering) (fill in your own answer).
- If another woman looks better than I or has nicer clothes or jewelry than mine, it bothers me. (Let's be really honest here!!!)
- I feel my best when someone compliments me on my appearance and feel bad when no one notices how I look.
- Others would think I was more attractive if I were (thinner) (more shapely) (bustier) (better dressed) (shorter) (wrinkle free) (_____).
- I would not want to be seen in public without my (makeup) (contact lenses) (fashionable clothing) (fine jewelry) (_____).
- I buy clothing and jewelry that I do not particularly like, because who am I to question the fashion experts.
- I could not have fun at a party or other social event if I were dressed differently from the other women guests.

Go back and assess each answer. Your responses indicate where other's "oughts" dictate how you look. As you go through the following chapters, look for ways to take back control.

One sees how [authentic] persona development for women as the first step in the individuation process is what I have come to call a desert experience, a time of going away into herself, all alone, perhaps for a very long time, in order to simply tune out all other voices and images other than the ones that derive from her own soul.

—Robert H. Hopcke, *Persona*

Five

Among the Ashes: The Appearance Maze

Alone, stripped of her former clothes, and dressed in a bedgown and clogs, Cinderella was made to work hard. Each day she got up before dawn to carry water, light fires, cook, and wash. On top of this, the stepsisters threw peas and lentils into the ashes and forced her to sit and pick them out again. At night, Cinderella slept by the fireside in the ashes. Each morning she went to her mother's grave and wept bitterly.

It's time to turn our full attention to Cinderella and explore the young heroine's role in our life. For her story is our story, and to successfully challenge the narcissus complex, we must meet her, see her plight as our own, and weep with her.

At the beginning of our life's story, we're like young fairy tale maidens—innocent girls, residing in our parent's house. We believe that if we're good and look like Daddy's little princess, princes will want us, and we'll live happily ever after. Even if our actual girlhood was far from a

77

story book world, cultural myths held that beautiful maidens grow up to become queens. So we do what's expected of us while looking as we "should." After all, doesn't the parlor-game rule say that if you play fair and look the part you will win?

I imagine that Cinderella, too, expected to grow up to be happy and successful. After all, her father was wealthy, and her mother was graced with innate love and beauty. Alas, however, her mother dies, leaving Cinderella with only a vague promise that God will take care of her and the mother will stay near by. But instead, Cinderella finds that nothing is the same any more after her father marries a woman who hates her and has two daughters who abuse her.

In our lives too, something inevitably comes along and shakes our world—like Cinderella we discover the fallacy in believing that if we play by the rules, we will win. But rather than winning, we experience a coming apart in midlife. We end up divorced, someone we love dies, or we lose our job, send our youngest child off to college, or have a serious accident or illness. Then again, we may begin to cry for no apparent reason. We soon feel unable to go on with life as we have in the past but have no clue as to why or what we can do about it.

When it comes to how we look, just as our bodies seem to betray us by aging beyond the acceptable standards, we see one too many teenage waif-models who look like third-world refugees blankly staring at us from the magazine rack. Or we hear one final inane decree from the fashion industry such as when Bill Blass told *W* that a woman can "forget it" if she isn't "skinny." Then, like the protagonist in the movie *Network*, we get mad as hell and aren't going to take it anymore. In this regard, our culture's obsession with youth fuels what comes next.

Regardless of how the shift begins, the results are the same for all of us. We dream of events, places, and people we thought were buried in the past and wake up feeling that something is unfinished. We daydream about the what-ifs of decisions we made long ago and try once again to justify the outcomes. Moreover, we attempt to answer illusory questions about our life's purpose.

What we're tripped into by this urge to reassess our past is called the midlife crisis, or more benignly, the middle passage. Being shaken into the turbulent waters of self-doubt is the first cue that it's time to turn inward—to seek the Self of which Jung spoke. For just as a child must grow into a maiden and then a matron so that she can take her place in the world, we must also mature from matron to crone in order to reap the harvest of the second part of our life.

But this is no easy task. Individuation involves reconnecting our egos to our Self and spirit, those aspects of us that society denigrates most and which we separated ourselves from when we banished our internal Cinderella to the kitchen in favor of the parlor. As Jungian analyst Marie-Louise von Franz writes, "The largely neglected archetype of the feminine in Christian civilization destroys the whole process of individuation, and the whole problem has to be rediscussed from those angles."

Indeed it does! Even though our souls have a new and different agenda as we reach our mid-years, our parlor-based ego fiercely clings to the world of glittery baubles and power. The late wisewoman Helen Luke wrote, "The ego will endure the worst agonies rather than one moment of consent to the death of even a small part of its demand or its sense of importance." So it becomes necessary for modern women to be *forced* onto the road toward individuation.

Banishment

If we view Cinderella's story as a metaphor for our midlife quest for individuation, we begin to see why it's necessary for her to be banished from the parlor. Although we're not told in so many words, we assume that before her mother's death, Cinderella's life consists of blissfully sitting in the parlor wearing beautiful clothes, much as Kore gathered flowers with her friends. This is akin to our early years of living in the heady material world of youthful fashion, intriguing relationships, fast-paced careers, and ego-enhancing possessions.

Given a choice, maidens would rather stay put—Kore and Cinderella in their idyllic surroundings, and us in the material world. But staying isn't the way of individuation. Over and over in myths, maidens such as Kore fall into some kind of peril that pushes them into the Great Crone's under-world. There, the wise older woman takes the maiden hand in hand and grooms her for her next stage.

But things are different now. Although the crises in life still present opportunities for us to make the inner journey, Hecate's realm is no longer considered the natural place for growth. Instead, when Hecate raises her lamp to light our way into our innermost recesses, we react to her as we would a banshee who tries to suck out our life's blood and drag us into a swamp. This is why in more modern fairy tales such as "Snow White" and "Cinderella," the crone is a witch or stepmother who cruelly banishes the maidens rather than assist them. In *She*, Robert Johnson describes the trauma we feel at the onset of our midlife call to transforma-tion as "a sort of inner chaotic evolutionary warfare."

Thankfully yet ironically, the evil fairy tale crone is still the one who ultimately facilitates the same teachings as did Hecate. By forcing maidens out of their father's parlors into kitchens, deep sleep, or forests, the older woman fosters transition on them. Needless to say, the maidens don't see this as positive, but it certainly is timely in their life cycle. Similarly, our life crises force us out of our ego-centered world and into a place we don't want to go. Yet, as with the maidens, if we honor the process we ultimately fare better for the trials and tribulations that such crises bring.

The Kitchen

Cinderella was banished to the kitchen, and the kitchen is also the metaphorical place of transformation in our inner self—the Great Crone's iron cauldron, where the ingredients of rebirth are brought together. The kitchen further symbolizes the laboratory of the Renaissance alchemists, metaphysicists who tried to transform base metals into gold because they thought gold was the *prima materia* of the Self.

Since our task in the kitchen is similar to the alchemists—to burn off the slag that chokes our golden Self and its spirit-based beauty—the steps in our mission are the same as the stages of the alchemical process: the *nigredo*, the black stage wherein we dissolve away erroneous beliefs and habits; the *rubedo*, where we become red hot with enough anger to make needed sacrifices, and the *albedo*, the white stage when we emerge from the cauldron transformed into a new being.

To move into the *nigredo* we must sever ourselves from our outer world so that we can die to our old ways. And make no mistake, separation from our material existence and reliance on parlor fashion is paramount, because we can't cut the bonds to our previous ways of dealing with life by remaining attached to them. Historian Lambros Kamperidis maintains that "It is only by retreating from the community and distancing ourselves from it that we come to an understanding of ourselves and our potential. This understanding brings about a transformation of our old selves, previously defined—ill-defined perhaps—by the community which gave us our identify, and this transformation allows us to realign ourselves to the world beyond the confines of our community and to rediscover our place in it."

Given that our appearance, above any other aspect, has publicly defined who we are for the past so many decades, it's doubly important that we move out of the parlor and into the kitchen. We can accomplish this by various means—meditation, depth analysis, contemplative solitude, reading books, and attending workshops, and retreats. I chose a combination of these, often relying on the expertise of women group leaders and authors who had traveled the road before me to show me the way.

Fear of the Kitchen

Regardless of the methods we use to help us move away from the parlor, the moment we hit the kitchen stairs we're gripped by unmitigated fear—fear of what might happen to us if we let go of our former reliances and defenses, go deep within, and really learn what we're capable of being. Cinderella's story points out why.

When we remind ourselves that the story speaks of how the various archetypes play out their roles in us, we see that although we may intellectually understand that our midlife mission is to reconnect to our Self and thereby rediscover our Cinderella-like spirit-beauty, our ego still resides under the roof of the wounded father. And since he and the stepmother have no desire whatsoever to assist us, we're like lost little fairy tale maidens who wander in the forest alone.

If you were ever lost as a child, you know the panic of rounding a corner and losing sight of your mom or dad. It's the same with first being in the kitchen. Nothing looks familiar, and you're scared out of your wits. Even knowing that your goodly Self waits for you provides little comfort, for when you're lost, even kind strangers can look ominous. And at this stage, the Self *is* a stranger.

Since birth we've believed that our packaged appearance is the only self we have, so in these early stages of the chaotic *nigredo* searching for our genuine Self is akin to looking into a mirror in the house of horrors. The Self appears ghoulish. We're no more able to imagine the joy we'll find in a spirit-based authentic appearance than Cinderella would believe at this point that she'll again wear beautiful clothes and marry a prince.

Turning Back

So we must be cautious. Our fear—our internal stepmother's most powerful tool—will tempt us to retake our parlor seat, to fall for ads for anti-aging creams and friends' insistence that a week at a spa will make us feel right again. "Do a little more waxing here, take off a few extra pounds there," they'll say. "When you look younger, your fears will go away." And for the moment, their suggestions may alleviate the inner call.

Anne, an artist in her mid-forties, was devastated when she was diagnosed with arthritis because she knew the havoc it could wreak on her career. But more troublesome, Anne associated having arthritis with getting old. It's as if her doctor had written "terminal old age" on her chart—a fate she wasn't ready to face. So rather than use the crisis as the push toward the kitchen door, Anne fled in fear and got a face lift.

But unfortunately, Anne's surgery won't mend her need to turn inward permanently. For the scenario of her inner story, and ours, still includes the orphan in the kitchen. No matter how hard we try to turn from our Cinderella selves we can't just sit in the public arena and drum her out.

Too, we must guard against our fear of the kitchen seducing us into believing that we're helpless victims. Yes, women have endured these many centuries of being forced to rely on a socially dictated appearance. In that regard, we *have* been preyed on by the system. But we only make things worse if we let ourselves become victims. Since victims feel powerless, and feelings of powerlessness already lie at the root of the narcissus complex, we who believe that we've been victimized are more likely to remain addicted to society's parlor image.

No, we simply must not remain in the parlor. As Helen Luke explained, "every time we are shocked out of some happy identification with another, which we have fondly imagined to be an unbreakable state, we are beset by the temptation to this surrender, to this despairing search for that which has been lost, demanding that it be restored to us exactly as it was, without any effort to discover the meaning of the experience. If we imagine we have succeeded in restoring the status quo, then the whole story will begin again and repeat itself endlessly and pointlessly until we can follow the goddess to the next step—the dawning of her attempt to *understand*."

Here again we can take our cue from brave little Cinderella. Instead of demanding that she be returned to the parlor in all her former splendor, she remains in the kitchen, even if it seems unjust, unexplainable, and unnecessarily cruel. So we, too, must stay in the kitchen and sleep in the ashes, the symbols of purification, of atonement. For by the ashes on her bedgown we know that Cinderella goes into the deepest part of her unconscious each night where something is at work, and as we lay by the fire of introspection, something works on us, too—the chaotic sloughing off of the *nigredo*.

And what of our fears? Psychologist Susan Jeffers, suggests, "Whenever we take a chance and enter unfamiliar territory or put ourselves into the world in a new way, we experience fear. The trick is to feel the fear and do it anyway." So we must face our fears, however great they be, and stay on our midlife path toward our authentic Selves.

Undressing the Self

As you approach the door to the kitchen, you may ask why it is necessary for Cinderella to be stripped of her clothing. For by now you know that Cinderella's story is your story and that you're about to have your dresses and shoes taken from you.

Prophets and poets from Lao Tse to May Sarton have written of the necessity of giving up in order to gain, in our case, to grow. So we who stand on the cusp of Hecate's crossroads, where one path leads to individuation and the other back to the parlor, must be severed from the most powerful symbol of who and what we have been—our inauthentic parlor appearance.

In having her dresses taken from her, Cinderella is stripped of her former identity as the innocent maiden. In sacrificing her shoes, she's left bereft of the naive premises she stood on during her early years. Indeed, clothing is so symbolic of who we are, that rites of passage since the beginning of time have included ceremonially removing one's former clothes.

As part of my work to free myself from the parlor's hold, I, too, made some changes. I put a diamond ring that my ego had been particularly attached to in the safe, along with a couple of other items that symbolized wounded power to me. I quit purchasing designer clothing and nixed my plan to have some cosmetic surgery.

These decisions were hard. Although necessary, letting go of that which had kept me afloat was still difficult because setting aside my former ego boosters left me bereft of a large part of my identity. One night I became so distraught that I asked Great Spirit "Why? Why is it that we must forego the blush of the early rose so that we can successfully walk into our second half?" That night I had the following dream:

I'm in Austin driving along Town Lake in my old luxury-model sports car that I called Foxy. I turn off the street, and the road becomes a rutted prairie trail that dwindles to no trail at all—just grass and sod. An icicle-looking mountain made of sand looms ahead. I rev Foxy but can't make it up the mountain. I wish I were driving Green Bean, the 4x4 Explorer I currently drive, because it could easily make the trip. Instead, I slide back down, and Foxy turns into an old flat-bed wooden trailer with no wheels. A bird dog with a bleeding left paw stands in front of me; behind me stands another with her left paw broken. I can't reach either dog, and they can't get to me because of their injuries.

This dream answered my question. I lived in fast-paced Austin during the 1970s when I was young and full of promise. Foxy's cool gray and sleek lines provided the perfect vehicle for getting me where I needed to go while I was on the public streets of my early years.

But my dream journey took me off the spring-green street, and I entered an open prairie that looked much as the unbroken Great Plains must have appeared to the pioneers. Prairie sand was formed by primal seas—the symbol of the Great Mother who's now as dried out as her ancient oceans. As I was raised on the prairies of West Texas, the setting also symbolized traveling back to the eternal feminine of my genuine Self, especially since the prairie evolved into a mountain—the ancient symbol of the higher calling.

I couldn't make it to my destination, however, because the car I was driving had the wrong *body*. I needed my current, less-sleek but better-equipped for off-road driving Explorer—the appropriate vehicle in which to bring potential life to the arid prairie and mountain.

Hecate's hounds stood before and behind me, just as she went before and behind Persephone. But since the dogs' left (feminine) paws were injured when I slid down the mountain, and I was now in a wheelless trailer, I couldn't reach them. Neither they nor I could do each other any good.

Other than telling me in no uncertain terms that my youthful body was not engineered for my upcoming season, the dream didn't answer specifically *why* it can't continue to serve as my vehicle. The full answer remains part of the Great Mystery. But the dream helped place my former appearance in a manageable context as something that would halt my journey, injure the Great Crone spirit in me, and render it inaccessible. Thus I took courage and continued on my quest for authentic appearance.

Lentils in the Ashes

Simply knowing that our former appearance won't do in our upcoming season doesn't give us a clue about positive aging, however. The Self is still too much a stranger at this point for that. So just as Cinderella works hard, so must we—scrubbing away our erroneous notions about who owns and controls how we look, washing ourselves clean of the belief that our worth is measured in carats and youthful beauty, lighting the fire of understanding of our Mother's beauty, and carrying water to our parched Self.

But how do we do these difficult tasks? Once again Cinderella's story lights the way.

As if Cinderella hasn't worked hard already, the stepsisters throw peas and lentils into the ashes and demand that she separate them back out. Here again, Cinderella isn't alone among maiden heroines in being assigned seemingly impossible sorting tasks as they toil in the *nigredo*. Baba Yaga made Vasalisa the Beautiful sort poppy seeds from dirt and good corn from mildewed corn, and Aphrodite forced Psyche to sort out a pile of mixed seeds.

That this sorting usually involves seeds of some type is no accident. Seeds are dormant potential that must return to the earth before they can sprout and flower, just as the maidens themselves must go into the underground of the Great Crone before they are reborn into a new phase. That's why it was so significant in my dream that the vehicle I needed but didn't have was named Green *Bean*.

In most tales, the seeds are mixed in with other material. The ashes into which Cinderella's peas and lentils were thrown symbolize purification. So once again we see that she's participating in the crone's mystery rather than a mere thankless task. While to all the world it looks like the Dark Mother's aim is to trip up the maiden, she is in fact testing her to see if she's worthy of transformation. For to sort seeds, a maiden must develop an understanding of what is and is not important, what should and shouldn't be kept, what can and cannot be digested—the very wisdom that the maidens will need in their upcoming season.

So it is with us. As our goal is to let our genuine Self shine through an authentic appearance so that it can empower rather than nullify the promise of our second half, the only way to grow this new type of beauty is to separate our appearance's good seed from its bad. And the only way to certify that the seed of how we will look in our upcoming decades is good is to purify it from all contamination.

But just because sorting is necessary doesn't make it all that easy. No, Cinderella spends long hours sorting out her piles. And like her we, too, have a great deal of work to do. Before us sits a mound of jumbled-up ideas, assumptions, and expectations about female appearance that have plagued women for so long that no one is counting any more. More likely than not, each has affected us in very a personal and perhaps vicious way—so much so that we might not even want to look at the mountain of seeds. Yet if we expect to journey on, we have no choice but to sit down and sort, knowing that somewhere in all this mixed-up mess lies a kernel of golden truth that will undergird our positive aging.

As we begin to sort, we discover a pattern of paradoxical themes that recur time and again in our lives and cast shadows over our appearance. Our task is to sort them into individual piles so that we can begin to get a handle on them.

Pile One — *Beautiful is Good / Beautiful is Evil*
My granny often quoted the nursery rhyme,

> *There once was a little girl who had a little curl*
> *right in the middle of her forehead.*
> *When she was good she was very very good,*
> *but when she was bad she was horrid.*

I've no doubt that she had good reason to repeat the rhyme to her curly haired, strong-willed granddaughter. But society's belief that beautiful is good is far more than a children's poem, it's a mandate right out of the father's parlor. That those who are beautiful must also be good—that is passive, deferent to men, nonaggressive, and dependent—is a *threat*.

The crux of the message in this pile is that although we must be beautiful, we shouldn't profit from our looks. Our beauty is for others—to bolster men's careers and egos, entertain others, help other women become beautiful by being models or beauty counselors, or sell cars, cigarettes, and beer.

If we use beauty for our own ends, we jeopardize the system, and run the risk of scorn. For example, successful and attractive businesswomen are routinely accused of sleeping with the boss, whereas less-attractive ones are assumed to have merited their successes. The wicked, attractive female executive who "pushes" her way up the ladder by being as assertive as her male counterparts á la Faye Dunaway in *Network* and Sigourney Weaver in *Working Girl* has replaced the evil stepmother in modern tales. The irony, of course, is that these assumptions demean *all* women, not just the beautiful.

As if these assumptions weren't injurious enough, this pile has a back-side. Women who make themselves attractive according to society's standards are often then accused of copping out to the system. Those who stay at home are called Barbie Dolls and Stepford Wives. Those who dress fashionably for their professions are put down because they don't look more like men. But of course, when a woman performs well and wears masculine-styled suits, she's called a butch. If she looks more feminine, she's labeled a bitch. Talk about a double bind!

This blatant put-down of women who operate out of their own convictions and dress to dance to their own tunes is worthy of a twelfth century monk. And if that's some people's intent, we who seek to create authentic appearance must not allow them to shame us into their ways

.

Pile Two — *Woman as Friend / Woman as Enemy*
We want only beautiful women in our parlors, yet we compete among ourselves for the spoils of victory—men. This woman-against-woman competition drives a wedge between us, yet paradoxically brings us together. Too many of us choose our friends as carefully as we would select from a rack of designer dresses at Marshall Field's, but that changes when men come into the picture. Here, the beautiful, particularly younger woman is the enemy, even to equally attractive women. So we learned early on to ease beautiful—and young—friends out of the way when a man enters the scene.

We also spar with other women in the political arena over the issue of female attractiveness. Many feminist writers express grave concern about the evils of the beauty industry, and rightly so. But in their attempt to divulge Seventh Avenue's sins, they also display disdain for beautiful women. Even within the women's movement the scorn of attractive women festers like an open sore, with Gloria Steinem too often negatively cast as the "pretty one." Yet we all must admit that she probably gets a lion's share of publicity simply because she *is* attractive. This is a sad commentary on both the movement that seeks to lift us out of our ills and the wounded society it targets.

In *The Beauty Trap*, a book that discusses several paradoxes which also show up in our seed piles, author Nancy Baker says she's *glad* she wasn't a pretty teenager, her point being that attractive teens often don't develop other talents. And that's true. But to be self-congratulatory for having not been an attractive teenager so that she developed other abilities creates a "good and ugly us" versus "bad and pretty them" schism. I cannot agree with either her logic or her methods. We must find a way out of this dichotomy by rethinking our notions about the meaning of female appearance—especially our assumptions about youthful attractiveness—so that we don't remain entrapped in this either/or beauty box.

Pile Three — *Beauty Is the Facilitator/Beauty Is the Stumbling Block*
As a society we assign traits of intelligence, creativity, and mastery to attractive children. Study after study show that teachers, parents, and classmates assume that good-looking kids are gifted with all the other positive qualities also. And guess what? It becomes a self-fulfilling prophesy. If we're told that we're brighter, more creative, and better able, we react accordingly (a good thing to remember when dealing with kids—or anyone, including ourselves).

But attractive young girls often find that at some point they're discouraged from using their budding talents. Rosa, a beautiful fortysomething woman whom I met at a seminar, sobbed and told the group how in her large Italian family the girls were expected to accomplish, but not to succeed. The boys, however, were expected to do both. So she put away her abilities and concentrated on being pretty and catching a husband. When her husband died at age thirty-nine, she felt despair at not ever having cultivated her own talents.

According to a *Los Angeles Times* article on the toy industry published in 1996, things haven't changed much since Rosa's childhood. Games for little girls, "focus on one element: boys. There is occasional reference to a career, or being smart, but the overriding theme of these and other girl games is that a girl should be pretty, plot how to get, keep or trade a boyfriend, go shopping, gossip, paint her toenails and her face, and kiss, kiss, kiss."

Rosa's experience and this article point out the crazy-making ambiguities in this pile of lentils. The message women too often hear from the wounded masculine rings loud and clear: "Be beautiful for me, but don't compete with me or better me in any way."

Quite simply, our culture views female beauty as an end all and be all. Beauty, it seems, gets everyone's attention, but then beauty is held to its position in the parlor—you're not supposed to *do* anything with it, just sit there. We're then reluctant to look beneath a woman's attractive exterior. And furthermore, we don't feel any need to. This becomes especially troublesome as our potential to accomplish increases in middle age.

As psychologist Robert Hopcke writes in *Persona,* "patriarchal sex roles are set up to devalue women and trivialize their selves and their activities, resulting in women's assigned social roles often embodying nothing but the superficial and trivial, for example, fashion and decorating, mere ornamentation designed to aesthetically enhance men's lives, and one has the situation in which many women sometimes have never experienced themselves except as the persona of a persona."

As if it weren't sinister enough that attractive women aren't taken seriously, we find that as we age, we're taken less seriously because we're *not attractive enough.* The double bind in this pile is beginning to look like a chaos loop. But it's true. Even as our abilities peak, we're not taken as seriously as are younger, more attractive women in our jobs, on the streets, at restaurants, and unfortunately for some of us, in our marriages.

And here, again, the media leads the way. A good example is one of Chicago's top female TV newscasters who confided to close friends recently that she's a face-lift away from being relegated to the back room. Any day now the windy city viewers will turn on the evening news and find that this talented woman has been replaced by a thirty-year-old. What's worse, few to none will complain of the injustice.

Pile Four — *Beauty Is Necessary / Beauty Is Vanity*
Society admires, copies, envies, and upholds beautiful women as the standard. But then it swats them on the hiney by calling them vapid, vain, and self-centered if they like and enjoy their looks, even the least bit. *Shame on them!*

Can you imagine supermodel Beverly Johnson telling *Mirabella*, "Yes, I'm beautiful. I'm just grateful to God that I'm one of the most beautiful women in the world today." This self-satisfied line of talk is encouraged in a running back who's just won the Super Bowl, but unlike professional male athletes who also spend a great deal of time readying their bodies for the game, any indication that we're *proud* of our appearance, or even that we are *pleased* with it, is verboten. Only the beautiful but wicked queen asks, "Mirror, mirror?" and then accepts the answer that indeed, she is the fairest.

I recall being shocked some years back when Dr. Joyce Brothers referred to herself as an attractive woman in one of her books. To me, a woman who was saddled with a narcissus complex the size of my home state, it was unthinkable that a middle-aged, professional woman would state publicly that she is attractive. Yet even after these many years of trying to rout my complex, I was teased by a good friend as she read through an early draft of this book. "Look," she said, "you refer to yourself as a 'fairly attractive' woman. You're not 'fairly attractive' you're *attractive*."

Egg on my *attractive* face!

We're in a real double bind here. We're forced to rate ourselves against other women's attractiveness. But when we do, and seem to fare well, we must keep it to ourselves. Again, we can't win the wounded father's game. Furthermore, this censure becomes doubly difficult as we age, because, as I've pointed out, we're not "supposed" to be attractive at forty or fifty, unless we've taken some fairly drastic measures to keep ourselves looking young.

Pile Five ⸺ *Beauty is the Symbol of Child / Beauty is the Symbol of Woman*
Were beauty merely the symbol of the feminine, our relationship with it might be less problematic. But according to society it's the symbol of the child *and* the twentysomething woman. At its most contradictory, standardized beauty bespeaks of the freshness and naturalness of a child who hides a sultry temptress. The '60s offered up Lolita and Twiggy; more recently Brooke Shields and Kate Moss took over the leads. Regardless of the decade, however, society seems to prefer infantile beauty.

The thought of an adult woman drenched in her own body odor, with hair streaming down her back in soppy strands and denuded of cosmetics, ravaging her lover sends shivers down our collective spine. Of course, what is scary about this all-natural woman is that she is experienced, capable, and savvy—a type of beauty that society isn't ready to accept. And it doesn't.

Instead, society shows us over and over on the silver screen that too much of what my college girlfriends and I referred to as "pure raw sex" in a woman brings downfall, loneliness, and destruction. Femme fatales invariably end up scorned, converted, banished, or dead, like Glenn Close in *Fatal Attraction*, whereas child-women ended up martyred, like Michelle Pfeiffer in *Dangerous Liaisons*.

In the late '60s the book *Fascinating Womanhood* instructed millions of us in our teens and twenties in the fine art of presenting ourselves to our husbands (no lovers or significant others in *this* book, thank you!) in a childlike manner. We pre–sexual-revolution maidens were taught that women should seduce with innocence and remain unaware of their bodies as they make love—to let sweetness and light cast a shadow of control over our passion. And although others of us who travailed puberty in the seventies didn't receive written instruction on how to mask our appetites in lamb's clothing, the cosmetic industry took up the slack. Such metaphors as babying our hair and pampering our skin left no guesswork.

What we don't take into account when we assume a childlike demeanor however is that children are weak, helpless, needy, and dependent because they're untried, incapable, and unknowing. Cute in kids, but where does that leave us as we move into our Demeter (much less Hecate) years?

The answer we get is that to remain alluring, we must create the image of never having lived. Or, if we've lived, at least that we've been sheltered. It's an affront that we've overcome obstacles and accomplished a few things, and as a result that we're wrinkled, roughed up a bit, and complicated-looking. So we're lured again into always looking like a maiden so that we won't offend the wounded father who fears our innate capabilities.

Adding to our quandary, many of us find as we age that our sex hormones don't wane with the brown in our hair. In fact, for the first time in our lives, we may be ready, willing, and able, as the saying goes. For despite the lid being placed on female sexuality, the primal sexual energy that surges through our middle-aged bodies increases after menopause. And this isn't some watered-down, latent-adolescent sex drive, even though we're expected to keep on looking like dewy teens. It's a demand for deep, meaningful, woman sex—the innate yearning of someone who's in charge of her own body, who can get what she needs from her lover, and knows how to return it back ten times over.

Yet while our hormones are saying "yeah, yeah, let's go wild," society is making us believe that unless we look and act like the Princess Bride, we have no right to slip into bed with the prince. Unfortunately, when it comes to who gets heard and who gets tuned out, too many of us lend an ear to the external "shoulds" that shame our midlife impulses into silence.

Pile Six — *Beauty is Natural / Beauty is Attained*

The oft-used fashion term *natural beauty* is an oxymoron if there ever was one. If you don't believe it, just look through any woman's magazine and see just how natural the editors really think a woman is without their advice and the products they advertise. Even Helen Gurley Brown reportedly admitted that the cover girls on *Cosmopolitan* are so average looking before the stylists and photographers get through with them that they aren't recognizable on the street.

There's nothing natural about packaged beauty, we're produced from head to toe—subcontracted out like a construction project. We wear makeup, our outfits must be put together, and we're told to create the right look. To appear natural we must color and artificially remove or add curls, paint our faces, work out the right muscles, and lose weight. When this fails due to age, we're candidates for laser surgery.

But, of course, our beauty must *appear* to come effortlessly. Like the secrecy that shrouded the ancient rites of female mystery cults, we must not talk about making ourselves beautiful or let anyone see us doing it.

Unlike other creative endeavors where the agony is 90 percent of the ecstasy, the common diet has no such class. Yet, our well-crafted appearance is on display for other's enjoyment the same as a Picasso or a Rembrandt! And while fine artists are congratulated for their time, money, energy, and pain, our grooming is the butt of a national joke. You can tell it's been a slow news day when the late night host starts his monologue with, "Today I spent so long waiting for my wife to get ready . . ."

Because we're expected to be parlor-perfect women, we aren't allowed the luxury of looking natural, not ever. Just looking like ourselves is so scary that some women don't dare come down for morning coffee without first putting on makeup.

A woman who lived across the street from my girlhood home offhandily told my mother one day that after five years of marriage her husband had never seen her in hair rollers (stock beauty aids in those days). It seems that she put them in each night after he went to sleep and took them out each morning before he woke up. While her need to hide her grooming activities seems a bit extreme, it isn't isolated by any means. Thousands of us have felt the pinch to maintain society's standards but are then shamed into hiding the fact that we change ourselves.

Katherine, a former colleague in her early sixties, often said that she wasn't interested in how she looks—that her childhood friends kidded her about her lack of interest in clothes. Yet Katherine's hair is never out of place, and her clothes are well-chosen, fashionable and expensive. One summer Katherine took a long vacation by herself and came back minus her wrinkles. Yet, she denied having a face lift, even to her closest friends.

Denial? Protest? Self-deceit? I don't know what drove Katherine. But suppressing her face-lift is underpinned by the same fear that drives many women to lie about their age. In one way or another, we've been collectively forced into duplicity in an effort to salve our feelings of unworthiness.

I'm not suggesting that our latest perm should be the main topic of discussion at next summer's company picnic. But women who hurt deep down often feel shamed into remaking their bodies. Then they deny it, because they don't want to expose the awful fact that they aren't perfect.

This also explains in part why society often shames the rich and famous when they remake themselves. We demand perfection from these women, but when Hillary Clinton gets an updated hairdo, the press castigates her. We don't want to be reminded that those in the spotlight are imperfect and need improvement any more than we want to admit it in ourselves.

Oh, what a tangled web!

Pile Seven — *Beauty Is The Treat / Beauty Is The Trick*
Since society maintains the belief that catching a husband should be our primary goal, it would seem that attractive women would have the edge. This assumption has led to the belief that the beautiful are more potent sexually, have better sex lives, and enjoy sex more than their less-attractive sisters.

However, this is another time when the Hollywood version of the fairy tale runs aground. While Prince is most likely happy as a clam with his beautiful new wife, Princess may find that life in the royal bedroom isn't that great. The strenuous dieting that Princess does to maintain her twenty-four-inch waist (not all that easy, given that most of our best-known fairy tale princesses are of Germanic, Slavic, or Celtic heritage) reduces the amount of sex hormones stored in her body.

To add insult to injury, after a life of making ourselves beautiful for others and being shamed if and when we thought that our bodies might be ours to please, it's not easy to satisfy our own sexual desires. So we take care of our partners and lay our needs on the bedside table along with our nightie.

The backside to this paradox is that in the *real* dating market, beautiful women are often overlooked. Although men may say they dream of dating a centerfold bunny, most wannabe playboys are too afraid of rejection to ask one out. So more attractive women sit home alone than we might suspect.

Then, on the other hand, when attractive women *are* sought out, they can never be sure whether they are loved for themselves or merely for their beauty. This question mark hangs over their feelings of self-worth like thick smog. The tragic lives of great beauties, such as Marilyn Monroe and Grace Kelly, attest to the fact that the more beautiful a woman is, the more vulnerable she is to becoming a victim of the very quality that makes her in such demand.

The Sacred Seven

It was no accident that there were seven piles of appearance-related lentils to sort, although I had no specific number in mind as I began to write. Seven is the sacred number of transformation. The Seven Sisters of Ursa Major were named for seven priestesses who founded ancient oracle shrines, and they carried over into Gnostic tradition as the seven caryatids associated with Sophia, the Mother of Wisdom. The Seven Hathors of Egyptian tradition were the wise women who met the dead in the afterlife and decreed their future. In Native American tradition, seven is the number of personal dreams—those nightly images from the unconscious that enlighten us as we journey.

Yet after trying to sort through our seven piles we may not feel enlightened, for the piles don't appear to supply us with guidance as to *how* to handle the disturbing information we now see so clearly. Thus those Seven Sisters of Wisdom look more like wicked witches.

But rest assured. The Seven Sisters *are* wise, but they are also illusory. Along with bearing wisdom, they protect against outsiders finding out their secrets. So it seems that even though we sit in the kitchen and sort through the piles, we're not ready to know the full truth. We're still strangers to our Self in too many ways. And to be sure, our unconscious holds more than we can or should know at this point.

Weeping at the Grave

Each day Cinderella goes to her mother's grave and sheds tears. Like her, we may weep hot, briny drops over the loss of connection between our appearance and our Self. Then too, we may weep in frustration. For me, the heat of menopausal night sweats held no candle to the bewilderment I felt as I lay awake wondering what I could really *do* about my inauthentic appearance. Although I was aware of the danger of being ensnared by the parlor during my autumn season, my ego appeared hopelessly dependent on it.

I reminded myself of my friend who had yelled at me about what we might come out looking like if and when we ever did emerge from the kitchen. It seemed as though I had only two ways to look—fashionably young or like an aging bag lady.

Yet if we truly want to move into the full splendor of our second half, we must allow our feelings and questions to come forth even when we have no idea of the outcome of our journey. Our distress and frustrations are to be expected, because the emotions that should have surfaced when we buried our inner Cinderella were covered over along with her. Now that we've rediscovered her, they are bound to pour forth.

In our determination to rebirth the long-lost maiden in us, let's take courage from the wise council of analyst and author Marion Woodman who urges us not to let the fear of the death pangs to our old ways hold us back from experiencing them simultaneously as transformative birth pangs. For truly, both processes are working in us at the same time.

Burying the Past

Some women find it helpful to create a ritual wherein they let their youthful looks die a natural death, mourn for what was, bury it, and turn away from their past looks toward their new life. Take a photograph of yourself at whatever age you feel you were your spring-green best. Look at the photograph. Remember yourself as you were then and bless yourself at that age. Then either bury the photograph, complete with a little box and flowers or ceremonially burn the photograph and scatter the ashes in a sacred place. Allow yourself to feel the loss, grieve for it. Then know deep in your heart that you haven't really lost the young woman you were, just as you know that the memory of a beloved grandmother or pet is still a part of you. As you turn to go, ask the spirit of the girl you once were to go with you as you move into the next phase of your life, and she will. She'll be there to remind you to take time to question, to see the good in life, and to have fun.

In nature, woman is healed from her weary
quest in the arms of Gaia, the original Mother.

—Maureen Murdock, *The Heroine's Journey*

⚊ Six

The Twig:
Autumn's True Raiment

Cinderella's father was going to the fair and asked his stepdaughters what he should bring back for them. "Beautiful dresses," said the first. "Pearls and jewels," answered the second.

"And you, Cinderella? What would you like?"

"Father, break off the first branch that brushes against your hat on your way home."

So the father bought beautiful dresses and jewels for his stepdaughters. On his way home, a hazel twig tapped against his head and knocked off his hat, and he broke off the branch for Cinderella.

When he got home, the father gave his stepdaughters the finery they had asked for, and he gave Cinderella the twig. Cinderella thanked him and took it to her mother's grave and planted it. As she wept, her tears watered the branch, and it grew into a beautiful hazel tree.

Cinderella sat beneath the tree and wept and prayed three times a day. Each time, a small white bird sat in the tree, and whatever Cinderella wished for the bird threw down.

We're not surprised that the stepsisters ask the father for finery, and that he buys it for them at the fair. But something more than parlor-business as usual is at work here. The Medieval trade fair included a carnival, where night after night bawdy, masked revelers in outrageous costumes danced and paraded until dawn. Then at midnight on the last night the costumes were removed in preparation for the high holy days that followed. Still today, Mardi Gras and Carnival goers remove their masks late on Fat Tuesday in preparation for the atonement and purification of Ash Wednesday.

So we see that the father's trip is much more telling than might be assumed at first glance, for once the gaiety of the fair is over and he travels toward home, a shift toward the sacred is at hand. And sure enough, the father's hat is knocked off by a hazel twig. In bringing home the twig for Cinderella, the father facilitates a transition.

By Cinderella asking for a twig, it would appear that being forced to stay in the kitchen sufficed to sever her from her former desires for finery. Yet let's not assume that by asking for a humble branch, Cinderella accepts her role as a scullery maid. Far from it. In asking her father to bring back that which knocks off his hat as he travels through the woods, Cinderella affirms that she wants life and all that life contains, but the life she seeks is *green* life—filled with spirit—not one hidden under the hat of the family patriarch. Cinderella further affirms her desire for this new life when she plants the hazel twig on her mother's grave.

Tears of Transformation

Although Cinderella wants life, she still has mourning to do. But now when she sheds tears, they produce tangible results. No more dark nights of merely searching among the ashes. Her tears go deep into the earth and bring forth a beautiful hazel tree, the ancient symbol of hidden wisdom and divination.

The tree, of course, is the symbol of life. Jungian Marie-Louise von Franz describes it as "human life and development and the inner process of becoming conscious. One could say that it symbolizes in the psyche that something which grows and develops undisturbed within us, irrespective of what the ego does; it is the urge toward individuation which unfolds and continues, independent of our consciousness." And in asking for the twig Cinderella *is* oblivious to her stepsisters' desire for dresses and pearls. Instead of parlor glitz, she craves the life-giving wisdom hidden in the hazel tree.

It's the same for us. One morning after we make the commitment to stay on the inner path despite our misgivings and questions, we again rise up out of the ashes, wipe the soot from our faces, and go to our mother's grave. *This* morning, however, we sense a difference. Amid our tears comes the cooling knowledge that we can do it—that we *can* stay with the journey even though we have no idea how it will turn out. And not only that, we *want* to stay with it because we intuit that creating authentic appearance is somehow life promoting.

My close friend Elissa, who is on her own midlife quest, came into my office one day and said, "I'm starting to cry up huge chunks of me. Even during the middle of the day I cry up pieces as though they were breaking off from a glacier deep inside me."

I looked at her, smiled, and said, "Good." But rather than protest what might have seemed a rather cavalier attitude about her tears, she said, "Yes, they are good. They feel *good*. I can't believe that I could cry like this and feel so good."

No more bile, no more hot and salty. These new tears are cleansing—baptismal. The chunks we bring up are pieces of our hardened emperor-like hearts that finally broke when our maiden-like tears fell, seeped in, and swelled up within it. And in their place, we make room for the wisdom-filled hazel twig to thrive within us.

Even though I didn't notice it as clearly as did Elissa, when I first let go of some of my fears and frustrations of what my authentic appearance might look like and began to trust the process, something shifted within me, too. For it was at the point when my tears turned from acrid to clear, pure, cleansing water, that I first tapped into the well-spring of my Self. Then it became clear why the vehicle I needed in my dream was named *Green* Bean.

Journeying to Mother

Similar to Cinderella's twig and the proper vehicle in my dream, our psyche now seeks to be made green. In days of old, women lived close to the green earth. They planted seeds and gathered fruit. Their cycles were one with Mother's moon. They tended their animals when they gave birth, and when it came their time, they squatted and let their blood run into the rich earth and brought forth life within and among life. When their monthly cycles waned, they sat quietly at Hecate's feet in remote, scared places and learned from her through the council of elder women. Then they rose up, powerful and wise, and took their place among them, just as Cinderella's hazel twig became a mighty tree.

But women's green ways eroded as they were moved from village to city in the name of progress. Sacred stones were overturned and places of quiet sanctuary were paved over in the name of development.

Most modern women today are too surrounded by steel and concrete to feel any real connection to the earth. And we who still live among trees and open fields no longer view nature as holy; even our sacred moments are enshrouded in man-made parlors. As mid-century writer Mable Dodge Luhan said, "Most of us are used only to the awesome holiness of churches and lofty arches, cathedrals where, with stained glass and brooding silences, priests try to emulate the religious atmosphere that is to be found in the living earth in some of her secret places."

To reclaim our connectedness to Mother's earth, we, like fairy tale maidens, must leave our homes and journey to the woods, desert, shore, or mountains. And like them, we must go alone and in reverence. This is no spring-break ski trip with the kids where conquering the slopes only adds to our conviction that Mother Nature is there for us to subdue. No, we must leave the idea of master and slave at our doorsteps and join with Her, hand in hand, Mother to child, teacher to student.

Obviously, I'm not the first to acknowledge the value of reestablishing our ties to nature. Listen to the story of any enlightened woman and you'll hear a similar tale. But although my personal story of going into the woods is far from unique, it serves as an example of how far the parlor is from our ancestral home, because I'm a prime example of the adage: It takes one to know one.

I "discovered" nature in 1989. I was a forty-two-year-old full professor and head of a university department. That year I'd taken students to Europe for a three-week field-trip, presented a research paper to an international group of marketers in Singapore, and then spent another couple of weeks in Asia visiting alumni and recruiting students. Throughout it all, I'd kept my appearance up with the best. To pay for trips to Beverly Hills for haircuts and the payments on my department store cards that taxed my regular paycheck, I taught extra classes at night and on weekends. Oh, yes, I had it all in 1989. I also had chronic depression, two severe cases of the flu, and shingles down my left hip and thigh—my feminine side.

Late one Friday as I hurried out of the faculty center, my secretary took me by the arm and said, "I hope this week-end you'll stop to smell a few roses." Trite? Yes! But true. If ever someone needed to smell the flowers, it was I.

So I took her advice. I walked, let my mind go, and looked at the flowers, trees, and birds in my neighborhood. I went to Malibu at sunrise and watched the rocks behind me cast purple shadows on the water's edge. I thought about who I was and what I was doing to myself. And I sobbed as though my heart would break wide open—which it did.

It would be several more years before I associated the narcissus complex and the facade it creates with women's failure to individuate, but during my hours and days in nature it became clear that something had hold of me. A false image of who I "should" be and how I "should" look was running my life.

The next summer Bud and I bought a cabin in the San Bernardino Mountains, and I learned what it means to be lonely in nature. As I said earlier, solitude is the enemy of we who are entrapped in the complex. But despite the loneliness, solitude at this point is paramount. von Franz writes that being alone is "the only way to heal the deep split and hurt. Collective standards do not help." We must first "reach the zero point and then in complete loneliness find [our] own spiritual experience."

Not only did I get lonely in the forest, I got scared, too. Nights in the mountains come early, and when there is no moon, they are black. Yet moonlight brings out the four-footed hunters, those who howl and run so close to my window that I can hear their heaving breaths.

But the fear of being alone subsides, for nature is our real home and our place of healing. After a day or two I realized that nothing was going to get me. What's more, I could feed myself, tend to myself, and make my own decisions. In a few more days I began to like it. After a week, I wondered how I ever lived without solitude's quiet freedom. Now I'm at my best when I steal away, alone, up to the cabin. Rather than lie in fear, at night my spirit races out the open window to join in harmony with the coyotes down by the lake.

Solitude's most valuable lesson was that it taught me to *listen*—to the birds, the wind, and even the overwhelming silence. We waste our efforts if we walk along the beach and drown out the roar of the salty billows with a Walkman or the voices in our heads—those ongoing tapes that tell us we're no good, others are no good, and life is no good. By listening to nature's sounds instead, we shut off the endless "shoulds," and let our Self wash us in Her quiet essence.

Autumn's Promise

When we quietly listen and watch, we learn of the nature of beauty and the beauty in nature. An old proverb says that the rose doesn't try to become a chrysanthemum, and the raven doesn't try to become a hawk. This is a good lesson. We humans pride ourselves on being the only rational animals on earth, yet we are the only animals who change our appearance in order to look beautiful. Rational? You tell me.

We learn about authentic beauty as nature teaches us about the goodness of each arc in our life cycle—another lesson women lost when moved from the rural trail to the fast lane. For as surely as the seasons and subseasons of the oak tree outside my cabin window revolve one into the next, our own autumn heralds not a death but a resurrection. How else could it be? The Creatrix who made everything else so perfectly cyclical wouldn't have made us any other way. It makes no sense that we, alone, would be born to blossom early and then spend the rest of our life merely withering away.

We in our mid decades stand ready to come into the most powerful and satisfying phase of our life because now is our season to reach in and realize our full potential. When viewed from this perspective, ours is a season worthy of celebrating. We should all join hands and dance in the streets.

If we observe the oak, we have good reason to rejoice. For it appears that she saves her best hues for October. No more pale green of spring or that tired drab of summer's end. She flames in reds and golds, sending color shock-waves against the azure sky. Indeed, our most vibrant time is upon us, too, if we but allow our leaves to turn fiery in autumn.

Midlife beauty is gutsy. It's knowing. It's intense. My midlife friends are an impressive bunch for the most part. They are deans and vice presidents. They write books and put together one-woman shows. Many raised fine daughters and sons and now look with renewed vigor at dreams, education, and professions they laid aside two decades ago. And those who allow themselves naturally to grow gold with October are *beautiful*—both in their countenance and in their bodies, because their authentic appearance is full, rounded, deep, meaningful, and personal.

The Mother Tree

In going to her mother's grave and mourning and praying, Cinderella makes her mother's story her own. By regenerating it and giving it a place to grow in her own life, the green that Cinderella wants so desperately sprouts from her mother's grave in the form of the hazel tree. And by actively working to grow the tree, Cinderella demonstrates that she's no idle bystander in her soul's transformation—she's a working partner.

Watering, weeding, and tending the grave of the Great Mother will bear green for us too. Just as with Cinderella, we cannot expect Her to open up to us without us doing our spade-work—getting our hands dirty and carrying our share of water.

When we put ourselves fully into our task, the tears we shed penetrate Her fertile soil in our hearts, softening and readying them so that She can work there. When we weed out erroneous beliefs about our parlor image, we leave clean fields where She plants seeds of self-discovery, understanding, and compassion. When we commune with Her in silence and awe, we open the portal of our soul to Her voice and tune our ear to Her message, for the hazel tree symbolizes divination—knowing through intuition—one of the Great Mother's most powerful tools.

Rest assured. If you go to the tree you *will* find the Great Mother. I cannot predict your individual circumstance, but when you reach the point of seeing that your former reliance on an inauthentic appearance has strangled your goodly Self, when you realize that you can never go back to your former seat by the parlor fire, and when you have prepared your heart to receive Her, you're blessed with Divine assistance. Just as Cinderella is nurtured by the white bird, you're met by a personal spirit guide who sustains you as you travel.

Often, as in the story of Cinderella, a bird becomes the intermediary between our human fantasies, imaginations, and potentials and the Divine. Birds, especially white birds, symbolize the Great Mother. Indeed, Her dove was transformed into the symbol of the Holy Ghost. And today, we who feel the presence of angels get a glimpse of them when we watch a white bird take flight.

The close association between angels and white birds gave rise to the alternative version of Cinderella's story where a fairy godmother befriends her. This Christian interpretation of an angel-like fairy godmother is preceded by an even earlier association between the white bird and Demeter. So there is a strong tradition of the spirit of the good mother coming to help her daughter, whether in the form of a bird or a fairy godmother. Thus we see that indeed, the dying mother's promise bears fruit. For by Cinderella staying good and pious, God *does* watch over her, and her mother stays nearby.

Animal spirits other than birds sometimes also enable those who quest for Self. We who search in natural settings according to Native American, Aborigine, or other traditional ways are often joined by an animal, either physically or in vision or daydream form. Such women may be befriended by female bears or wolves as they meditate—symbols of the ancient feminine, whose wise and fierce motherly instincts know exactly what it takes to raise us, their cubs, into mighty she-bears and she-wolves.

As with Cinderella's white bird, spirit animals give us whatever we ask. So if and when we request guidance, we'd better be prepared for the answer and the animal's way of answering it. For although Mother is loving,

She has a mission—to get us ready for our second half. So it's no child's game we play when we knock on Her door and ask to be let in.

This was certainly true for me. As part of my study of Native American traditions, alone on a craggy mountain side during a vision quest, I laid with my stomach flat to the earth and prayed to Great Spirit for guidance. After some time, I rose up and faced north, the direction of animals and wisdom. No sooner had I stood than I heard a rattle and went numb with fear. Where I grew up in West Texas people don't think of the dry rasping of a rattlesnake on a moonless night in the middle of nowhere when you're a quarter-mile from base camp as the voice of the Great Mother.

But then I remembered my task. I'd asked for transformation, and the snake was my sign—the oldest symbol of Gaia's transformative powers lay coiled in front of me. I knew in my heart-of-hearts that if I truly believed in what I was doing, I'd be safe. With that, the snake slithered away, leaving me with a physical sensation in my heaving chest as though something was leaving my body. In what amounted to no more than a few seconds the snake taught me more about the primal feminine than I could have learned from a mountain of books.

Returning to our Roots

That Cinderella's tree thrives means that it put down roots. And for us to realize positive aging, so must we.

We put down roots by turning to women who've walked the journey before us. Jung suggested that we go back five or six generations to find our blood-related roots. And the roots of our full female heritage lie even farther back, for we are products of *all* women who've gone before us. Since most of what we need to know is stored in our deepest memories, finding our roots is as simple as merely tapping into them.

While Hecate may seem a mere ghost from the past whom I've

brought back as a metaphor for learning how to age, she isn't. She's as real in the underworld of our psyche as she is in Persephone's. And many women are finding her through deep meditation, guided visualization, and in dreams.

In *Revolution from Within,* Gloria Steinem wrote a detailed description of how she met her inner wisewoman and of the things she learned from her. I was impressed with her candidness. But for such openness with one another, we would trudge along the backroads of our journey alone, thinking that our experiences don't happen to anyone else, and that perhaps we're either possessed or crazed.

I met my wisewoman one night as I meditated and let my imagination run free (a process called active imagination). I found myself in a most primitive, round-shaped ceremonial hut that was lined with furs and baskets. Simple tools hung from the ceiling, up out of the way of a circle of women and animals seated on the floor. After I joined them, a gray-haired medicine woman in white deerskin and turquoise and silver jewelry appeared. Her skin was wrinkled and brown like a walnut, but when I looked into her eyes, they were as clear and blue as a mountain lake. She came to me and painted my face with sacred colors, thus bringing me into the council of women. Over the years Ancient Grandmother has appeared spontaneously, and I can call on her as needed, just as Cinderella calls the white bird. Other women find that as they open up they are guided by angels, light, or simply overwhelming feelings of nurturance and warmth.

At or about the same time I met my inner wisewoman, I became interested in studying Native American tradition. It called to me as I drove across the desert on my way back to Texas from Los Angeles. I recalled an incident, long forgotten up until my interest re-surged. When I was about six, I told my family that I was an Indian—much to their amusement. For my button nose and green eyes bore no resemblance whatsoever to those with whom I claimed kin. Then some two years after I began my studies, I discovered that indeed I am part Cherokee, by way of my maternal grand-mother—a fact that had been swept under the dust of the family tree early on. But the truth finally surfaced, as truth does when we're open to it. Since my maternal lineage is part Cherokee, it's no accident that my internal wisewoman is Native American.

We may also be drawn to a heritage or deity that's not traceable in our bloodline. I was born on Hecate's day, the twenty-second of October, and I am truly Hecate's child—partial to the underworld and brooding on the mighty impact the unconscious has on our lives. But then, of course, we're all related to all wisewomen whether they originated in Anatolia or Africa, Polynesia or Peru.

Women may also hear a call from their more immediate female heritage. Carol spent several years researching her matrilineal heritage—a monumental task given that her grandmother had been an orphan. When Carol had uncovered her roots as far back as possible, she recorded her family tree in a book that she gave to her mother as a present, along with a trip back to the site of the Georgia plantation where their family's first American matriarch was born. There, in the dark Georgia dirt, Carol and her mother wept for joy as they honored their foremothers.

The Grandmother Tree

That Cinderella's tree was a hazel tree is significant. Hazel trees bear nuts—dormant states, entombed in womb-like shells while they lie in rest under the earth until it's time to sprout. In this, nuts have long been associated with the crone. And given that hazel trees, in particular, have long been associated with divination and ancient wisdom, their connection to the crone is doubly obvious.

But the death-before-life arc in the ongoing cycle of life doesn't just involve the crone. Underworld transformation also incorporates the young, unborn state within the nut who benefits from being so near the source of wisdom. That's why in the earliest mythology, Persephone and Hecate were one-and-the-same goddess. Only later did they separate into the patron goddesses of granddaughters and grandmothers.

I cannot over-emphasize the need we have for grandmother wisdom during our transition. Whether our own grandmothers were able to impart special knowledge to us or whether we must seek it from other village grandmothers, we are desperate for what they know. For in beholding the grandmother-tree and ingesting her wisdom, we encounter a glimmer of the love and acceptance in our Selves.

For many of us our grandmothers were our refuge—the ones who loved us unconditionally. Others of us may have had a kindly older neighbor, an aunt, a family friend, or a teacher who loved us simply because we were who we were—no strings attached. If we relive our memories of these women and again experience that warm, safe, feeling we will know once more what it is like to be loved simply for ourselves. That's how we are loved by our Self.

Since grandmother wisdom incorporates the knowledge of our innate goodness, it stands to reason that it also holds the key to positive aging. So the next step in our journey is to mine the Self for this ancient knowledge.

Journey to the Self

By going to her mother's grave three times a day and weeping on it, Cinderella makes it lush with the ancient feminine. Three is the number most often associated with the maiden's journey, the only number with greater power than seven. In Native American tradition, it resides in the south—the direction of sacred plants and the innocent child who quests in wonder. According to British mathematician Keith Critchlow, number three completes the sphere, giving it an interspacial quality and the ability to contain. A better description of the integrated feminine couldn't be found in an ancient manuscript—for the primal feminine's womb from which all springs is the sphere: whole, composed of inner space, and above all, containing.

I believe that we, like Cinderella, profit from making three pilgrimages into our unconscious during the quest to divest ourselves of our inauthentic parlor mask. So I include three guided visualizations—techniques for tapping into the unconscious and dealing with the information stored there—in the seminars I teach.

During the first session, the women meet their inner child at about the age of nine or ten, for she is the one we must heal first if we expect to bridge the ego and Self. Often, on introspection we find that as young children, we were happy, carefree. We played ball, climbed trees, read, played with our dolls, or just hung out. But rarely were we troubled about the way we looked. All that changed, however. Invariably, women report feeling both a loss of innocence and the onset of the appearance-based complex sometime around age nine.

Visualizing our inner child at that age often proves excruciatingly painful. For example, Dolores' chubby inner child refused to look into a mirror—a necessary part of the visualization I take them through that shows each woman how her inner child feels about the way she looked at that age. As a child Dolores' classmates had called her names and picked her last for teams, leaving this part of her hurt and ashamed. Unfortunately, Dolores' inner experience is common. Even as mature women, we find it difficult to "face" the appearance-related shame we received as children.

To mend these early hurts, we must go back to an even earlier time in our life, perhaps age two or three, before we severed ourselves from our inner Cinderella. Then we move forward again, but this time we provide a green environment for that precious little girl to live in so that she can thrive in an atmosphere of love irrespective of how she looks.

To help heal my inner child, I used a technique called active imagination, a similar process to guided visualization but where the imagination is set free rather than entrusted to an outside facilitator. I went into a meditative state and then let my imagination set up a scenario in which I visualized myself at each age in increments of four or five years from toddlerhood up to my early twenties. Then I imagined that I talked with myself at each age about beauty, accomplishment, and the true meaning of who I was and am. Then, before I moved on to the next age, I visualized hugging my inner child, teen, and young adult, just as I would a loved one in real life whom I was leaving. Although the task proved difficult at times, the results were well worth the pain, for it allowed me to reflect on my early years, the time when I was developing an inauthentic appearance, with compassion and love. In this way, I was able to heal at a very deep level.

After my seminar participants determine when and how their inner child was affected by society's parlor mindset, I lead them through a second visualization. Each woman's spirit guide meets her in a moonlit clearing and takes her to a sacred place where she meets her wisewoman, much as I met Ancient Grandmother. Then they ask their wisewomen to tell them about their genuine beauty.

This first brush with the primal nature of female beauty often provides the turning point whereby the women link their innate goodness with their physical appearance. And even in its brevity, the results of the encounter can be immediate and instantly transforming.

After being lead to a clearing by a brown bear and meeting a group of elder women, Nancy wrote the following in her journal:

The old women said to me,
You have raised a son.
He is now twenty-four.
He is happy and takes good care of himself
and loves himself.
He loves you very much.

You have taught him well.
Now you have arrived at the next part of
your womanhood.
You are a wise woman,
a free woman,
a loved and admired woman.
You can wear this flowing purple
dress made just for you.
It is soft and light and skims
loosely over your fullness.
You can let your hair be full of moonbeams.
You can let go the striking young woman
and be the beautiful wisewoman with
moonbeams in her hair.
You can wear sandals that let you breathe
and walk surefootedly for miles.
Let the bear lead you back
to your clearing in the woods,
where the moon is full
and will light up your hair
and your eyes.

What a testimony to positive aging!

The third visualization is far less structured than the first two. After I take participants into a deep meditative state, each one simply asks the void what she needs to know about her authentic appearance.

Because the women have opened themselves up so profoundly by this time, the results are often overwhelming and sometimes just a little more than what they may expect—much like my night on the mountain. I've seen women become defensive at what they experience. Others become frightened. But I haven't worked with any who weren't touched deeply.

By now we know that the unconscious contains that which we don't often understand and may not want to. Yet we cannot skip the instruction that comes to the surface during the third journey, for it can provide our most necessary lesson. Three, after all, is the magic number that completes the sacred womb, the soul.

When I went in and asked for truth, I was first immersed in total blackness—far darker than any moonless night in the forest. And I, too, was scared. Within a split second, however, I was surrounded by colors unlike any I'd perceived with my human eyes—blues, magentas, yellows, greens, and violets. They rolled over me and through me like waves on a shore, again, and again, and again. I heard no voices, no songs—nothing. I felt only the surge of each wave towing me under with a power I can neither describe nor understand. And neither do I understand the goodness and acceptance that I felt. It asked no questions, it gave no answers, it simply swirled me in rainbow water that transcended anything I'd ever experienced. And to this day, I've never felt it again.

It's far beyond me to comprehend what I tapped into. Faith alone tells me that it was what I needed at the time, that it was good, and that it was right. And to be sure, it has taken time to sort through the message. Far better that our inner essence would tell us straight out in plain English what the heck it wants us to know and do. But that isn't the way of the unconscious. Messages come to us encoded in a mystery that is ours to perceive but not necessarily to understand.

I do know, however, that from that day forward, I never again viewed my aging body and all that it encompasses as a commodity, as belonging to someone else, or as being mine to harm if I so please. Truly, if my flesh can serve as the receptacle of power that mighty, that accepting and loving, it is a temple—a holy vessel that I must not desecrate for as long as it is mine to wear.

Finding the Path

Am I special, different from other women? Are my inward journeys unique? Absolutely not! Once we clean out our pipeline to the Self, each of us has the same ability to reach in, expand our souls and tap into the pool of the Divine.

Moreover, there's no right or wrong way to approach the Self. Certainly tried and true methods exist, attested to by great philosophies and religions that have withstood the centuries. But each belief system has its merits. It's up to us to determine the best route to Divine wisdom.

I only have two personal biases regarding how a woman travels the inner roads. First, I would encourage anyone to steer clear of any teacher, preacher, shaman, or psychologist who maintains that his or her way is the *only* way. I believe strongly that there is no one way, and given the myriad of backgrounds, heritages, levels of education, predispositions, and preferences that abound in women, anyone who claims to have *the* way is either misinformed or trying to generate a cult mentality.

My second bias is against any group that refuses to give women *primary* leadership roles and fails to acknowledge that women are powerful, good, and innately spiritual. These patriarchal notions and the groups who adhere to them negate the entire process of journeying in and finding the strength necessary to break the bonds of the appearance complex.

When we get down to it, however, it's really the spade-work we do in our own backyard that will get us where we need to go in our journey. Yes, teachers, masters, counselors, and authors, are helpful and can ease our process by showing us a few short-cuts and assuaging our fears. But the end result of our trip will not and does not rest on the amount of money we have spent, how many sacred sites we have visited, or the star-quality of our teachers.

Undertaking trips and signing up for seminars—even buying and reading books of this type—work best when directed by our inner wisewoman. She, the white bird, will let us know where to go, how to get what we need and from whom. That's her job.

Our job is to ask for Her guidance and then *apply* what She suggests, whether it comes through sitting under a tree in our backyard reading a book or from meditating on a mountaintop in Peru. Unfortunately, this application sometimes gets lost. There are some women who never apply Mother's lessons because they're hooked on the *process* of becoming. They go from one seminar to the next nonstop so that they don't have to process what they learn; or they keep the trails to the self-help shelves in their library hot, but never apply what they read. This is serious. Such women are said to have a Persephone complex. They prefer to remain in Hecate's realm rather than take what she teaches and use it in their lives. Robert Johnson writes in *She*, "To identify with the mystery is to lapse into the unconscious, which is the end of any further development. Many women who safely make the journey this far fall into the trap of identifying with Persephone's mysterious charm. No further development is possible to them, and they remain a kind of spiritual fossil with no human dimension."

So let's remember—Persephone only lived in the underworld with Hecate for three months each year. For the other nine, she lived in the upper world with Demeter and carried out her duties as a corn maiden. Our mission in life, too, is to live *on* the earth and *in* it—not to separate ourselves from it. Otherwise, why would we have been given these glorious bodies?

Bridging the Gap

For most of us, remaining in Hecate's realm is a nonissue. Even if we would like to stay a little longer sometimes, we have people to feed, jobs to go to, relationships to tend, and shopping to do.

Yet, moving back and forth between the unconscious and the physical world can be difficult. There were times when I first began my inner journey that I felt like I lived in two completely different worlds—and I did. Driving back down into the Los Angeles basin after being at my cabin for only a few days left my disposition as polluted as the air into which I drove. By the time I got home, I was either in a snit or on the verge of tears because the transition was too great.

Since spanning these two worlds is difficult at best, it's necessary that we build a bridge between them so we don't become fractured. Fortunately, three tried and true methods of bridging the conscious and unconscious have withstood the test of time: Creating a sacred space, creating art, and creating ritual. When it comes to clearing the deck of our appearance-based complex, we have no choice but to recognize and honor our need for all three. For they are the means by which we will ultimately unite our body, mind, and soul so that we can adorn ourselves in the authenticity of spirit.

Creating Space

We bring the sacred right into our physical world by creating a holy place for ourselves—a sanctuary. Up until now, our only sacred space may have been our dressing table, for upon it we laid our hopes, our dreams, and the full extent of our self-worth. But time has come to worship something different.

Women build altars by nature. Since the beginning of time, they have kept the hearth and the family shrine. In *Casting the Circle*, Diane Stein tells that all of us build altars in our homes, and it doesn't take long to spot one in someone's house if you know what to look for. By instinct we define an area as sacred and fill it with those things that have deep meaning for us, whether it be a collection of family photos on the piano, a wall of framed college degrees, or a handful of souvenirs on a shelf in our bedroom.

Along with countless others who expound the value of creating a holy space, I, too suggest that we clear a space for ourselves and fill it with those things that we hold sacred. It doesn't have to be large; a corner will do. But it must be ours and be respected by those we live with as being ours.

Women often place pictures of themselves as children on their altars. Others include rocks, shells, or feathers—natural objects—that have meaning. Some put religious insignia on their altars such as a medicine wheel or a Madonna. I have a friend who collects small statues of women in local costumes when she travels and has them arranged on her fireplace hearth. That spot is so compelling that first-time visitors invariably go to it instinctively.

Once we build it, we must spend time in our sacred place. It becomes our refuge, the place where we are closest to our spirit mothers and our ancestors. I sit at my altars at home and at the cabin to worship, think, and just be by and in myself. Since I spend most of my time at my office, I put together another small altar above my computer. It's amazing how many women *and* men comment on and touch my collection of things.

By sitting at our altars we remind ourselves that our bodies are good and lovable. We honor them as temples of spirit by involving them in our sacred moments when we relax, breathe deeply, refrain from poisoning them with alcohol, tobacco, and other drugs during our quiet times, hold our objects, smell the sage, incense, or candles we burn there, and experience the silence.

Tapping into Creativity

Anthony Storr tells us in *Solitude*, "People who realize their creative potential are constantly bridging the gap between inner and outer." The Self is the seat of our divine spark, our creativity. For when we were made in the image of God, the ember of creativity was placed within us. Thus our ultimate task in life is to create—to become aware of our unique talents as we journey inward and then bring them forth into the tangible world.

The word *create,* however, has taken on a meaning that's far from its original association with the Divine spark. We're so indoctrinated to believe that only those who are good enough to sell their art are creative that we don't dare pick up a brush and paint a picture unless our work ranks with Cézanne. But this isn't the real meaning of creating at all. When we bring that which is in our hearts into the world, whether it be a song, garden, or major project at work, *that* is creation.

When we explore nature, it's good to write about what we see and feel in our journals, create poems, draw or paint, take photographs—in other words, physically record what is going on around us. After each active visualization, I request that the women in my seminars first write about their experience, as did Nancy, who expressed the visit with her inner wisewoman so eloquently. Then I pass out art supplies.

I like to get out the crayons and butcher paper and serve juice and cookies after we've spent time with our inner child. Since we're already sitting on the floor, it doesn't take any time before these sophisticated women are giggling, borrowing colors from each other, and, for all the world, looking like a bunch of second graders.

But in every group one or two women balk. Some cry in frustration as they look at their empty paper. Then the stories pour forth about a teacher, parent, or sibling who convinced them at an early age that they couldn't draw. Imagine, telling a child that she isn't creative, that the work of her little soul isn't good enough—no wonder we grow up to feel that we must dress to please others and that the uniqueness in our aging body is a crime! For adorning ourselves is as much a creative act as picking up a Crayola. So to relearn how to dress in the image of our true Self, we must first relearn how to create from our heart.

There are no right and wrongs when it comes to creativity. Our unconscious holds a vast reservoir of symbols that are significant to us. And it's the personal interpretation we give these symbols that directs the authentic appearance we want to wear. Given that the meaning of our symbols is personal, who's to say who is better or worse at interpreting them? Joseph Campbell reassures us that "one should not be afraid of one's own interpretation of a symbol. It will come to you as a message, and will open out." *Open out*, I love that phrase.

This point about opening out was brought home to me in no uncertain terms when I took a workshop from ceremonial mask-maker Laura Denny where we made a plaster casting of our face and then decorated it. When my turn came, I closed my eyes and breathed deeply as Laura applied wet plaster bandage-strips to my face. As the warm strips molded around my features, I focused inward. Moving past sound into quiet, color turned to image. Further into my recesses, image gave way to the black void.

All too soon I heard Laura's disembodied voice telling me to unmask—jerking me up through the tunnel that connects subconscious with conscious. Dark became indigo, indigo became color, and color gave way to blinding incandescence. Still hanging somewhere between dark and light, I looked down into the dead-white impression of my face. Pasty, raw and in need of life-giving definition, the mask urged me toward paint and brushes. Yet fleshing it out was no simple task because it gave what seemed to be mixed commands.

The right side demanded sleekness and polish. I scattered small pearls across glossy, salmon-colored skin and edged the severe line of its uncoifed face with matching silk-soutache braid. As I worked, this side began to mirror modern sophistication.

I turned to the left side. No sleek paint here. It begged to be made moist and warm—earthy. A gritty sluice of red-ocher dirt from the spirit-filled hills of northern Arizona bathed its features. The unruly russet-brown hair cried out for shells and hawk feathers. Finally three turquoise-colored lines graced the left cheek bone.

Emotions pounded as I looked into the mask's finished features. Although the two sides were different, she looked whole—integrated. She was powerful. She was beautiful.

"Who is she?" Laura asked. "Where did she come from?"

As Laura waited for my answers, so did I. I was overwhelmed. Powerful, yes . . . integrated, yes . . . beautiful, yes. I was drawn to the mask's strong presence and sense of self. But she seemed only dimly familiar, and I didn't know why. Wasn't she born of my own face and hands?

That night I went to my altar and put the mask up to my face. As my eyes looked through hers into a mirror, a faint recollection shivered through me; then an epiphany. I'd known her forever but long ago had relegated her to my subconscious where she'd waited until I rebirthed her when I meditated in the black void.

The mask was the embodiment to me of *integrated* and *authentic* female beauty. The three turquoise lines on her left cheek recounted the eternal waters of life. Her feathers and shells were fetishes of the exalted, primal woman. And although modern, her polished right side sprang from her the essential feminine. Pearls, now looked on as trinkets of the elite, originally sang of the sea—primal waters—amniotic fluid. Her silk braid bespoke of mythic spiders' webs that connected heaven and earth.

Today she hangs on my office wall. And if I ever forget who I am or the meaning of authentic appearance, I look at her.

Creating Ritual

If we aspire to link outer and inner as symbolized in the mask, we must learn to create ritual—to physically incorporate our active visualizations and prophetic dreams into our tangible world by *acting* them out. Otherwise their healing messages will remain deep within our unconscious and have little chance of impacting our every-day lives. As Robin Heerens Lysne expresses in *Dancing Up the Moon*, "Whether we acknowledge the sacred daily or create once-in-a-lifetime rites of passage, the key to living a richer, more sacred life is moving from our hearts. Our hearts are the center of life-force in our physical bodies. The love in our spiritual hearts radiates from our soul and connects us to life."

In *Inner Work*, Robert Johnson describes ritual as a "physical *act* that will affirm the message of the dream," or visualization. "It could be a physical act . . . Or it may be a symbolic act—a ritual that brings home the meaning of the dream in a powerful way."

Just as I went home from the workshop and ceremonially put the mask up to my face, I suggest that my seminar participants go home and ritually reaffirm what they learned about their authentic appearance from their inner wisewomen. Some make necklaces and wear them when they meditate; others dance out their visions. This physical affirmation of inner awakenings drives home whatever point is made by the unconscious and helps translate it into a *physical* acceptance of the message. For it's not just our minds we're working with, it's our entire *beings*.

I suggest that you, too, celebrate the symbols of your heart, and thereby bring them into existence. If dancing or making ceremonial jewelry isn't your thing, bake a special cake and eat it while contemplating your heart's message. Or take a moment each morning, face the east, bring the symbol of your good Self to mind and hold it there while you stretch out your arms to the rising sun. What a way to start your day!

When we link body and mind to the unconscious through such rituals, the message seeps to every level of our being in a most profound way. When we pay special homage to the genuine beauty that our birds point out, those parts of us that are used to being told that they're not good enough are reprogrammed, thus moving us one step closer to bridging body and Self.

Returning to Mother

As we rush through busy schedules in our concrete fortresses, it's easy to forget that natural beauty isn't standardized. To relearn this primal meaning of beauty, spend as much time as possible each day alone, and observe nature—no friends, no book, no chatting with the other woman on the park bench. I don't care if you live in a high-rise in the middle of Manhattan, you can see something green each day. Eat lunch in the park. Those pigeons have something real to say about beauty. Their iridescent feathers glisten with every color in the rainbow. Yet they flock together irrespective their shining colors—blues, greens, whites, grays.

As you take your first steps out of the parlor, you can't spend too much time alone with nature. Even a long drive in the country will do wonders. If you can get away for a weekend, all the better. A longer nature "fix" is the best gift you can give yourself—but again, no husband, no odometer on your bike, or a race against your last MPH. Take the dog and *walk!*

When you go, go unadorned of your parlor best. Wear faded jeans and an old sweater (my idea of what we'll wear in heaven!). Let your scrubbed face be touched by the wind just as the father's hat was brushed by the twig. Squirrels don't care whether or not you have on makeup, and neither will you after you go without it a few times.

You'll discover that all things in Mother's world are both beautiful and unassuming. Chick-a-dees and daisies are oblivious to how the others look. Observe a field of flowers to see if you can find any two blossoms which are carbon copies of each other. You can't. And yet they are all beautiful.

The Inner Child: Visualization

The following shows you how to visit your inner child through a guided visualization, much as the women in my seminars visit theirs. Working through the exercise will help you feel the spontaneity that little girls feel before they are seduced by the looking glass.

Visualizations can work on many levels. If you aren't familiar with the concept, think of it as a daydream or a story in your head that relates to you on a deep, subconscious level. The good you get from it depends on how much you let go and take in what comes to mind as your visualization unfolds. So involve yourself in your visualization to the fullest by remembering the details, looking for colors, and experiencing any emotion that you feel. Remember three things as you start out. First nothing whatsoever can hurt you as you proceed through the exercise because you are in full control. Second, you can stop at any time. And third, your experience may differ from the script. That's okay because this is merely a suggested guide. Each of us reacts differently depending on our unique experiences.

I suggest that you prerecord the script and play it back to yourself or have a trusted friend read it to you so that you don't have to remain conscious enough to read while you complete the exercise. In this way you'll be able to free up your mind to get the most from your experience. Allow plenty of time between each line in the script so that your mind can set up each scene and follow through.

Choose a comfortable, safe place to sit or lie quietly. Allow about a half hour of uninterrupted time. Have your journal or a pad and pen read to use as soon as the visualization is over.

Relax and breathe deeply for a minute or two. Then turn on the tape or have your friend begin to read the following to you.

See yourself sitting on a park bench . . . Feel the sun warm on your shoulders . . . wiggle your feet . . . and settle into the bench.

Look up into the clear blue sky and notice the number seven forming in the clouds . . . watch it disappear . . . now the number six . . . watch it fade from your view . . . the number five . . . now a four . . . watch the number three . . . two . . . one

As the one fades, bring your attention to a group of little girls playing nearby . . . They look to be about four or five years old . . . Are they playing jacks? . . . skipping rope? . . . playing hopscotch? . . . pushing their doll buggies? . . . Listen to their laughter . . . Hear them squeal with delight as they play.

One of the little girls notices you and waves in recognition . . . Do you know her?... She may be someone you know or someone you have never seen before ... She may be you at that age.

How you feel about her?... Are your feelings about her good?... Do you like her? ... Good ... If not, choose another little girl whom you like and see her wave at you.

The little girl comes toward you ... What does she have on?... What color is her hair?... See the laughter in her eyes as she comes near ... She may say something to you ... When you feel like it, stand up and take her hand ... Hug her or greet her physically if you wish.

As you take her hand, notice that you have left the park ... She leads you into a special room or a place where there are lots and lots of wonderful clothes, and shoes, hats, ribbons, or whatever you wish. Maybe there is it an old trunk, or an oversized comfortable closet. Is it your room when you were a little girl?. . . Let her show you around.

Watch her as she begins to pull out pieces of clothing and try them on ... What does she put on first?... Feel her joy at touching the clothes and combining the colors.

Does she ask for help?

Do you wish to join her?

Let her choose something for you ... She may want to help you put it on ... Feel her little hands smoothing the folds or setting the hat just right.

Allow as much time as you wish to play with her ... You may want to play act, or have a tea party, or just look at yourselves in a mirror and laugh.

What do you see?

What do you feel?

What colors do each of you have on?

(Pause)

When you are comfortable and have played enough, take the little girl back to the park ... Be sure and thank her for letting you play with her wonderful clothes ... You may feel like telling her that you will come and play with her again ... If either of you feel sad at your leaving, make plans to meet again before the end of the week.

Watch her as she goes back to her play group.

Return to your park bench . . . Feel the hard slats against your back.

Look up into the sky . . . See the number one appear in the clouds and then disappear . . . Then see the other numbers appear and disappear in order up to seven . . . As you reach seven, feel yourself return into the room. Don't rush, take all the time you need . . . When you are comfortable, open your eyes.

Write down as many details about your experience before you have time to analyze it. By doing this you keep your ego from editing out the parts it finds troublesome and enhancing those that it agrees with. After you've recorded as much as you can remember, you can begin to reflect back. What was your inner child's relationship with her appearance? What emotions came up. Depending on the age of the inner child, you may have felt shame, as did Delores in the earlier example, or you may have felt your inner child's elation at being able to express her authentic self.

To make your experience more concrete, draw a picture or make something that reminds you of the visualization. Then create a simple ritual, perhaps taping the picture to your mirror and looking at it and reflecting on it each morning for a week. In this way you will bring the essence of your inner child and her apppearance to the forefront of your mind where it can help you heal.

Once we see that living up to our standards appears to be leading toward self-destruction, the time has obviously come to question our standards, rather than simply resigning ourselves to living without integrity. We must summon up the courage to challenge some of our deepest assumptions concerning what we have been taught to regard as the good.

—Nathaniel Brandon, *Honoring the Self*

Seven

Sorting:
Creating Authenticity

The King announced a festival that was to last for three days. All the beautiful young girls in the country were invited, so that the King's son might choose a bride. The stepsisters were overjoyed and called to Cinderella, "Comb our hair, brush our shoes, and fasten our buckles, for we are going to the King's festival."

Cinderella obeyed, but she wept, because she, too, wanted to go to the dance. She begged her stepmother to let her go. But the stepmother mocked her. "You go, Cinderella? You are dirty, and yet you would go to the dance? You have no clothes and shoes, and yet you would dance?"

But Cinderella wouldn't give up. At last, the stepmother said, "I have emptied a bowl of lentils into the ashes for you. If you have picked them out again in two hours, you shall go with us."

Cinderella went into the garden and called, "You tame pigeons, you turtle-

doves, and all you birds, come and help me pick the good into the pot, the bad into the crop."

The birds came into the kitchen and began to pick—pick, pick, pick—and gather the good lentils into the bowl in less than an hour. Then Cinderella took the bowl to her stepmother with a glad heart because she could now go to the festival. But the stepmother said, "No, Cinderella, you have no clothes and you can't dance. You would only be laughed at."

Again Cinderella wept. And the stepmother said, "If you can pick two bowls of lentils out of the ashes in one hour, you can go with us," thinking to herself that Cinderella wouldn't be able to complete the task.

But again Cinderella called to the birds. This time, they separated the lentils from the ashes in a half hour, and Cinderella took the two bowls of lentils to her stepmother.

If we had wondered about whether the parlor ego had been displaced as we slept in the kitchen and wept at the tree, we have our answer. The stepsisters are still up to their old tricks. And this time, they've really got something to get dressed for—the king's festival. Vain as ever, they demand that Cinderella help them get dressed—giving no thought whatsoever to the fact that she might want to go with them.

In our personal stories, too, our egos have no mind to allow our Self any say over how we adorn ourselves, despite our reawakening to the truth about authentic beauty. For our egos have lived in the parlor all their lives and are still calling the shots.

What *has* changed, however, is Cinderella's attitude. She wants to get out and dance, and she won't take no for an answer. No longer the cowering child, she confidently asks her stepmother for what she wants. And, after nights in the kitchen and days at the Mother's grave, we too feel a new desire to get out—to take what we've learned about our Selves into the world.

Just when we're ready to let our newly found Cinderella out, however, the stepmother reenters the scene and throws more lentils into the ashes.

And while the stepmother's reappearance may seem untimely, it isn't out of character. In numerous fairy tales, stepmothers, witches, ogres, devils, and murderous husbands reemerge just at the crucial point when the maiden seems for all the world as though she's accomplished her mission.

That the Dark Mother never fails to return at this crucial time points out the significant fact that finding goodness and love within our Selves does not eradicate the darkness. Quite the contrary. Discovering the light brings out what Jung called the shadow. For by all laws of nature, the dark *must* return whenever we turn on a light.

If you step outside on a moonless night, everything looks flat because you can see only varying shades of dark gray. But turn on a flashlight and you instantly set up a field in which the contrast between dark and light is striking. Those objects in the shadow appear even blacker than they looked when you had no light at all.

That's what happens to our psyche when we bring in the light of the feminine. Before, everything looked gray, murky, and unfocused. But just as soon as we begin to light up areas, shadows are also brought to focus. And the brighter the light, the more pronounced the shadows become.

So instead of merely dispelling the darkness, our newfound feelings of Self actually help us identify, explore, and integrate those split-off parts of ourselves that we've cast to the deepest shadow in our unconscious. This is vital, because what we are unaware of ultimately controls us, but when we bring these hidden aspects into the light, they can no longer have the upper hand.

Our appearance shadows may contain our need to make ourselves look better than other women or our beliefs that our aging tummy needs a tuck or our arms are too flabby. The list is endless. Regardless of what they are, at the bottom lies the fear that we're not good enough—that same old fear that keeps our egos in the clutches of the father's parlor.

But despite our fear, we, like all good fairy tale maidens, must deal with our shadows before we can adorn ourselves for the ball. For up to this point, we've had no opportunity to explore what to replace those old beliefs about our aging appearance with. Believe me, it's one thing to see how the errors of the centuries have entrapped us in inauthentic appearance, but it's quite another to reprogram them. When it comes to making drastic changes in our behavior, such as completely reimaging ourselves as we grow older, Kenneth Gergen advises in *The Saturated Self* that, "We cannot leap headlong into new vocabularies of being any more than we can speak a foreign language we have never heard."

So, as much as we might hate to admit it, the stepmother is right. We have no clothes to wear to the festival. And, when we look at it from this perspective, the stepmother's seemly vile behavior is a blessing. By repeatedly making us purify lentils—the embryonic premises from which we will create an authentic appearance—she forces us to sacrifice our old ways in favor of the new.

The Rubedo

Even though it might be for the eventual good, my guess is that Cinderella didn't want to separate more lentils from the ashes. But, by now, she is so determined to go to the festival that she's willing to do the stepmother's bidding. This willingness, however, brings her to the second stage of the alchemical process, the *rubedo*—the place of sacrifice, for she wants to go to the festival so much that she's willing to acquiesce and perform more tasks for the hateful stepmother.

It's the same for us. We want to take what we've learned at the Mother's tree and go dance so much that we're willing to sacrifice our desire to keep all the old stuff about aging and appearance hidden in the shadows. We're willing to take a look at it and sort the good from the bad, even if it means prolonging our desire to go dance.

This is a crucial step in our individuation, for it involves reassessing our life's course in relation to our old parlor image and making choices about how we look that will empower us to proceed with the purpose of our second half. And there's no doubt about it, if we don't face our shadows at this point, we cannot grow any further. By forcing ourselves to look squarely at our appearance shadows, however, we're motivated to take action to ensure that we do.

For example, Denise, a tall brunette in her fifties, traced her acute shyness back to being the tallest child in her grade school. Towering above the other girls as well as standing a half-head taller than the boys made her want to run and hide. As she describes it, "I wasn't a cute, petite little girl. I was big—bigger even than the boys. I could easily run faster and jump higher. But that wasn't an okay thing. So I slumped and tried to act like a little lady by sitting in the corner."

Now Denise is a well-respected dietitian, but she never outgrew feeling ill-at-ease around other people. She realizes that her decision to become a dietitian instead of the corporate lawyer that her heart desired so strongly was due to her preadolescent shyness based on her size.

When Denise analyzed her situation, she considered going to law school. However, she now loves her work as the senior dietitian for a large HMO. So instead of going back to college, Denise joined Toastmasters. She's hoping to use her commanding size and newly developed talent to make presentations to groups who need to know about good nutrition, such as women's shelters, schools, and day care centers.

While Denise made a major life decision circuitously based on the fact that her appearance didn't measure up to the other little girls, Beverly's situation was exactly the opposite. Her striking beauty surpassed most of the other girls at her high school.

Now in her early forties, Beverly told me how her high school counselor recommended that she try out for cheerleader during her sophomore year rather than play basketball as she had dreamed of doing since she was a child. As Beverly was both black and popular, the counselor felt that she would add a proper racial mix to the all-white pep squad. To coax

Beverly to his way of thinking, he shamed her by asking why a pretty girl would want to play basketball when she could be a cheerleader—the goal of most teenage girls in his opinion. His guilt trip worked, and she cheered on the sidelines for the next three years.

Even though outstandingly athletic, Beverly never got her chance to play varsity basketball. And she never got a chance to go to college, either. Although she admits that no one can know for sure whether she could have earned a basketball scholarship, it's for certain that she had no other means of affording a degree. Instead of going to college, Beverly married the high school football star the summer after they graduated, had the first of two children ten months later, and worked as a secretary while he played football at the local junior college. The marriage lasted less than five years.

Like Denise, Beverly has thought through the changes she wants to make. She has her eye on a position in the marketing department of the large entertainment-based corporation where she works as an administrative assistant. This new job will allow her to get dressed up and put her outgoing personality on the line. The only thing keeping her from taking the position is that it requires a college degree.

But Beverly's too wise to let a little thing like that stop her at this age. It seems that the company's benefit package includes tuition reimbursement. As long as she maintains at least a B average, they reimburse her for three-quarters of her costs. Earning a B in my consumer psychology course was no problem for Beverly—she finished with the highest A in the class.

In one way or another the decisions we all made early on in our lives are similar to Denise's and Beverly's. And to be sure, going back and reliving them in our minds can do nothing to change them. But attempting to change the past or shaming ourselves for it aren't the purposes of the three bowls of lentils. The object is to analyze how being female in general, and how our appearance specifically, played a role in the decisions we made along our life's path so that we, like Denise and Beverly, can adjust our attitudes, choices, behaviors, and appearance and go to the dance.

Yet because of the complexity of our relationship to our appearance and the degree to which it helped shape who we are, assessing its role in our life can be difficult. So let me assist you in three ways.

First, as you work through each bowl and reflect on what it has to say about your parlor image, be patient with yourself. You may need several weeks to come to any conclusions. We often don't connect life's events and decisions to our feelings about our appearance at first glance, because its effects are so ingrained, subtle, and pervasive that trying to isolate them is akin to looking for the forest as we stand in a thicket. So rather than being struck with insight immediately, understanding is likely to come in bits and pieces.

Second, don't fall into either/or thinking. Women are complex, paradoxical creatures. Our relationship with our appearance has been neither all bad nor all good. Too, judging the quality and texture of our life's decisions isn't as easy as putting them into neat little boxes labeled *good* and *bad*.

We've lived so long in a wounded society that much of what we might consider positive at the outset actually is no more than sugar-coated symptoms of the narcissus complex. For example, if one of the bowls prompts you to remember your high school prom because you spent the three or four hours basking in the spotlight covered in white tulle, you might want to delve into why you felt the need to hold the spotlight for so long and why your prom night, of all the events in your life, popped to mind.

I'm not implying that this experience categorically is symptomatic of the complex. But it could be. And if on examination you find that something you've deemed positive is tainted with traces of parlor mentality, you need to think about it for a while.

Conversely, what might appear to be negative at first may turn out to be a gem in the rough. For years, I thought my teenage obsession with making clothes was a symptom of my obsession with my appearance—that

I spent most of my free time and an inordinate amount of money on fabrics because I craved the fashionable clothing of my more affluent friends.

On further reflection, however, while my adolescent need to keep up with my friends no doubt motivated me, it didn't explain the hours I spent dyeing trims to just the right color, putting in handmade buttonholes, and combing notions departments looking for just the right buttons. It also didn't explain why much of what I made didn't really look all that similar to my friends' clothes or that much of it remained unworn.

Only after I took up watercolor painting several years ago and eventually had to find extra storage for my paintings—paintings that I do purely for self-expression rather than for decor or show—did it dawn on me: My teenage passion for making clothes was an *expression* of my Self— an act of *creation*. More importantly, it was the only outward statement a shy, self-conscious teenager would allow herself. Now, I thank the Creatrix that during my teens I had my creative drive, my fabrics, and my sewing machine.

Finally, although we have more sorting to do, *this* time when we tackle the bowls of lentils, we're not left in the kitchen unassisted. Cinderella goes to the garden, calls the birds, and they come. Likewise, we're no longer little girls who cower in the dark and wonder what on earth to do with all of the conflicting and injurious information about our appearance. We have birds to call on. We can trust our spirit guides, inner child, and inner wisewomen to help us make decisions about our appearance. So as you begin to work through each bowl, ask for help. I assure you, it will come.

Bowl One: "Shoulds"

By now we realize just how much of ourselves we've given up in order to maintain an inauthentic image. Our overwhelming need to please others by conforming to their *shoulds* results from the perversion of an otherwise normal process of socialization. Humankind learned early on that adhering to social norms was necessary if society was to remain intact. But the need for conformity in appearance metastasized somewhere along the way.

The truth is, even without the pressure of society's *shoulds,* few to none of us would break the rules to the extent that we would cause a scene. So don't worry that if you retake control over how you look and dress from your heart you'll come out looking incredibly bizarre or want to run naked in the streets. Rest assured, you won't.

To pinpoint the exact nature of women's fear of dressing from their hearts, I ask them to figure out where they can go without feeling that they must wear a perfected image—full-face makeup, the latest fashion, or whatever they feel they *must* wear. For some women the answer is, "Nowhere." Like the emperor, they rely on their perfected image from the time they come down to breakfast until they crawl into their nightgowns.

Even women who don't feel the need to look perfect all the time feel threatened by this question, because it asks us to state the extent that we rely on our parlor image. Furthermore, it asks us to look at ourselves objectively rather than subjectively. And we who feel the pull of the parlor are the least able to stand back from ourselves and question our motives and actions. For when we do, all the darkness in the shadow rises up within us, puts its icy hand on our shoulders, and tells us that we're not good enough to dance.

By forcing this shadow to present itself openly, however, we're able to shed light on it. I'm reminded of Donna, a woman I met at a group who was studying *The Beauty Myth,* who cried out one night while we were going over the questionable tactics of the cosmetic industry, "*I* don't even like to look at myself without makeup. Why would anyone *else* want to?" By the startled look on her face, I saw that this painful realization came up unexpectedly from the deepest corner in her psyche—the one in which she tried to bury her Self under the false assumption that she's worthless without a "fixed" image. Yet as agonizing as it was, her realization touched on the very assumption that she most needed to bring light and love to.

For many of us, the answer to the question varies, depending on circumstances—who will see us, and how we feel about ourselves at the time. During a particularly hard time several years ago when I felt just rotten about our finances, I answered the door and found two of Bud's business associates who'd come to pick him up for a meeting. I was a mess—no makeup, faded jeans, and an old T-shirt. I was so embarrassed I just stood there stuttering, afraid to look them in the eye until Bud rescued me.

Less than a year later we gave an informal supper for a few friends. In the rush to get everything ready, I forgot to put on makeup. It wasn't until everyone left and I went to wash my face that I discovered that I didn't have a whole lot to wash off. Rather than melt, I laughed and went to bed.

In both situations my feelings about myself made all the difference in the world in how I thought others would perceive my appearance. In the first, my low opinion of myself colored how I thought Bud's associates would think of me—unworthy. In the second, I was in good spirits. My life was going well and my inner work paid off by helping me realize that I didn't always need to wear makeup.

Can we say I was free of the appearance complex at the time of the party? Unfortunately the answer is no. But at least I was headed in the right direction, because if I had forgotten to wear makeup before I had begun the journey to reconnect with my Self, nothing could have kept me from coming unglued—not even winning the lottery.

This brings up another important question: Can we cure ourselves of the narcissus complex completely? Again the answer is probably not, because our society is so deeply afflicted with it. And we are products of society no matter how much we try to extricate ourselves from its dictates. But society's tenets must not stop us from doing what we can to lessen its effects. Our personal goal is to come as close as possible to believing that no matter what situation I'm in, I am a worthy person. My worth is not tied to my appearance, and I am not at the mercy of how others perceive me or how I think they perceive me.

Top Billing

A second issue in this bowl has to do with how important our appearance is to us, for at the top of society's *should* list is the directive that we make our appearance our number one priority. But, of course, we now know that giving our appearance top billing limits our other midlife potentials. To assess who gets the starring role in your life, ask yourself a number of questions: How often does my appearance crop up in my mind and conversations? How much attention do I pay to how I look? Do I routinely read fashion magazines, look at fashion ads in the newspapers, and shop for new styles? Do I ever forget how I look while I'm doing other things?

What a list of questions! Yet by answering them, you can see the extent to which your appearance is a priority, because they point out where you are expending time, energy, and money. And as I stressed earlier, whereever you spend these, so goes your life.

One of the clues that let me know that I was making headway on my complex was when I became aware that after I got dressed in the morning, I rarely thought of my appearance again. Just to check it out one day, I shut my eyes, and, sure enough, I wasn't even able to recall for a number of seconds what I had on.

Dependency

Given our goal to create an authentic appearance, one that reflects who we are at this stage of our lives, the third issue in this bowl has to do with who would be affected and how, if we didn't wear a perfected image around them. Nathaniel Brandon writes in *Honoring the Self,* "To the extent that we have successfully evolved toward good self-esteem, we hope and expect that others will *perceive* our value, not *create* it. We want others to see us as we actually are—even to help us see ourselves more clearly—but not to invent us out of their own fantasies. Even if the other person's fantasies concerning us are complimentary, we feel invisible, unseen; we feel unreal to the person who may be professing to adore us. In the responses of others, we long for *appropriateness*."

Here we assess where we may be caught up in others' illusions of who we *should* be. Depending on your personal situation, you might ask, "If I didn't wear makeup to the office, who would it affect?" Or ask, "Who would care if I didn't have on a new dress at the party on Saturday?"

Your parlor ego will be put on full alert by this question, because it threatens her. Then she, like the stepmother, will try to back you into a corner by telling you that you're going to end up looking frumpy, that you'll wind up making a fool of yourself, as well as those near and dear to you.

I can hear her now. "Not wear makeup when you make the most important presentation of your career? How stupid can you be?" That's an exaggeration of the question. Needless to say, you might want to wear makeup when making a public presentation.

"Not buy a new dress for your daughter's graduation? Are you crazy? A mother needs a new dress for such an important occasion." And your ego is right, you probably would buy a new dress for the graduation. But again, that's not what the question implied. So stay with the original question: *Who* would be affected if . . .

If we take our question to our birds and ask it without fear and the clatter of our ego, the answer for most of us is, "No one would really be affected." We would still be who we are, others would still be who they are, and life would go on.

However, if in asking the question you still believe from the bottom of your heart that certain people would experience some repercussions by your not creating a socially dictated image, ask yourself a very difficult next question: "Why? Why is this person or are these people so in need of me living behind a false parlor persona that my creating a more personal image would affect them?"This is a tough question because it requires you to identify those to whom your appearance represents a commodity, where you are being used to buoy up someone else's failing self-esteem, or where you have become enmeshed with others, based on how you look.

The realization that someone you love is dependent on your appearance plays havoc with your self-esteem. And disengaging the dependence calls for all the Self-affirmation you can muster. In her column in *New Woman,* Harriet Lerner offered some positive advice to a woman whose husband was critical of the twenty pounds she had gained since turning forty—advice that could be applied to any of us who find ourselves in a similar situation. First, try to learn as much as possible about his feelings regarding your changing appearance. What bothers him about your size (wrinkles, shifting hips, or whatever)? Is he embarrassed about it? Does it make a difference in your love life? How did he and his family relate to people who were fat or old or wrinkled, and how did they deal with it? Is he concerned about your health?

As he answers the questions, don't punish him for being honest, for we are looking for his authentic reactions. And be honest with him, too. Express your concern about growing older, gaining weight, or turning gray. Also express your new awareness about positive aging. For example, you might say, "This is part of who I am at forty or fifty or sixty. And I'm beginning to like me just the way I am."

Finally, if he doesn't respond to these positive means of dealing with your aging body, Ms. Lerner suggests that you tell him to back off—that he has a right to how he feels, but not at the expense of hurting you. Then explain that you will discuss your changing body any time he wants to, as long as it is in a positive, constructive manner.

But you must be careful before you come to a hard-and-fast conclusion that others, especially the men in your life, hold you responsible for creating the image they need and want to see. I've talked with dozens of men who are genuinely concerned with their wife's or girlfriend's concern with her aging looks. It seems that these men find their wives or lovers as appealing (if not more so) as ever and wonder what the fuss is all about.

So it may not be that others *really* are that enmeshed with your appearance at all. Your ego may be threatening you by overshouting the truth—telling you that your husband demands that you stay young looking, that your friends will abandon you if you don't look the same as them, and that you will be laughed out of the office if you dress from your own heart. The fact is, once we get past other people's *shoulds* we who dress from our own hearts look just fine, and we can dance with the best of them.

Validation

In addition to supporting our fragile ego with society's rules, we, like Snow White's stepmother, look into the mirror and ask, "Who's the fairest?" Yet, we're afraid to hear the answer, because it more often than not serves only to confirm the flaws we try so hard to mask. So, for we who are entrapped in the parlor, the mirror is both our ally and our enemy. We fear the poor image we might create without it, but we don't like what we see in it either.

While few women look into their bathroom mirrors and genuinely appreciate what they see, too many of us are incapable of acknowledging anything good the looking glass has to offer because of the *shoulds* that play like repeating tapes in our heads. How many of us stand before the bathroom mirror and look past our shiny hair and trim legs and find wrinkles around our mouth? Or we say, "Look at me, I'm overweight. My husband will run off with a younger woman" or, "How can someone my age go back to college? I'll look like the other students' mothers."

It appears that most of us need anywhere from a little work to a whole reprogramming to break the mirror's double hex. While I'm not a real fan of affirmations because I believe they can mask the underlying causes of our problems and push them deeper into the shadow where they cause greater havoc, I firmly believe that if we use them *after* we've uprooted the cause of a complex, they aid in our healing. So I now urge you to develop a limited number of affirmations.

All an affirmation needs to do is get the attention of your parlor ego so that you can begin to introduce her to your Self's way of thinking. Think of a word or a short phrase—*beauty, I'm beautiful,* or *pretty me.* Perhaps you prefer something more gutsy such as *gorgeous.* Be sure to avoid words that conjure up the image of a young girl, such as *babe, baby,* or *kitten,* or that of a sex object such as *luscious* or *tempting.* Remember, this is about affirming your authentic looks as you go into midlife and beyond.

For the next two weeks, say the word every time you see your reflection. Say it out loud if you're alone and to yourself when you aren't. And say it with *conviction*—Cinderella didn't whimper about wanting to go to the dance.

At first you may have to say the word again and again, louder and louder, because your internal stepmother will merely brush you off. Mine even mocked me a few times, "Oh, you're going to say that word *beauty* again." And I came right back and said, "You bet I am, *beauty!*"

Once you get comfortable saying your word to your reflection, begin to say it every time you have a negative thought about your appearance. Shout down those thoughts about wide hips and crow's feet.

Before long, you'll look into the mirror one morning and say to yourself, "Beauty, I'm beautiful," and it won't be a mere verbal affirmation. Then your soul will sing a little song all day.

Just Say "Thank You"

Even though we dance to others *shoulds,* too many of us shake off their compliments once we get the steps right. What irony! We're addicted to hearing other people tell us how good we look, but accepting their appreciation challenges our low opinion of ourselves so we can't take it in.

Instead, we blast innocent complimenters with every reason why they've made grave mistakes: "Oh, this old thing. I think it makes me look fat."

I like to begin seminar sessions by complimenting one of the women on how she looks, and then sit back and wait for the lesson to unfold. And my method to get the point across has never failed. Not once has anyone ever responded with a simple "thank you."

Although most of us are incapable of acknowledging compliments with a "thank you," that's how the Self would respond if we would but let it. So with a little practice this straightforward answer becomes automatic. And as with the personal affirmation, once we've accepted a few compliments gracefully, we begin to agree with our Self that we deserve them.

Bowl Two: Sacred Sexuality

As in days of old, our sexual energy is one and the same as our *creative* energy, what is known in some traditions as our *Kundalini*. Thus when we speak of midlife potency, we're talking about a lot more than just a romp in the bed. As our monthly blood begins to slow, our inner urge to fulfill our Selves in every way rises like Hecate's full moon on an October night.

As painful as it might be to wake them up and hear them howl, if we want to wrest out the promise of the rest of our life, we can't let the sleeping demons of our wounded sexuality lie in our shadow. We must bring our distorted sexual identities into the light, heal them, and return our sexuality to its place of honor. While it's beyond the scope of this book to delve into the full scope of our sexual wounding, three cultural myths about our sexual persona negatively impact women at midlife to such an extent that they must be addressed.

Myth One — *Men shackle women to the singular role of sex object and keep us from fulfilling other roles.*
It's time to face an unpleasant truth. Men aren't the only ones who fetter

us to the stereotype of woman as sex object. Despite women recently carving out new niches, too many of us still cling to old patriarchal beliefs rather than develop ourselves in other ways. I'm not blaming us for causing our plight. We didn't. I *am* suggesting, however, that it's time we drop the notion that women are mere decorated vessels.

Andrea, a professor in her mid-forties, is a flirt, a vamp who bats her eyelashes and slinks around in skin-tight dresses. Although married with two children, she comes on to every man she sees—professors, students, and her friends' husbands. Needless to say, the campus is ripe with rumors, and Andrea is the butt of jokes. What's sad about Andrea isn't so much what she is, however, but what she isn't. Her role as femme fatale is her *only* identification. I sometimes wonder what other traits and talents are overshadowed by her sexual persona. An artist? A good mind? Who knows?

Then there's Barbara, the wife and darling of Skip. Given half a chance, Skip will tell you about Barbara's sexual prowess. As he roars on about what a lucky man he is, she beams, blinks, and giggles like a teenager. In the many years I've known her, she's never let on that she thinks of herself any other way than as Skip's bedmate. Does Barbara feel the need to express any other part of herself? Does she harbor a desire to learn music or sculpt or, for that matter, carry on a conversation about a subject that she is particularly fond of?

Andrea and Barbara both act out the narrow role of a sexy woman, albeit from opposite perspectives. And while it may seem harmless enough, in reality, playing out this singular role smothers the Self. When we relate to ourselves *only* on a sexual dimension, we restrict the conditions under which we interact with both men and women, and we gag those rising needs we have for expressing ourselves in so many other ways.

No one is purely sexual. Even women who have a stronger sex drive or a more highly developed sense of their sexual image than the average are, nevertheless, other things, too. But when society casts the net of woman-as-sex-object, the Andreas and the Barbaras get ensnared, and then do little to free themselves.

We need to remember that sex is *good,* and that looking attractive to our partners is absolutely necessary to our relationships as well as a whole lot of fun. What I'm getting at, however, is that we need to be aware of the price we pay for creating a unidimensional sexy appearance.

Evelyn, the fifty-five-year-old owner of a small real estate agency, feels that she's paid enough dues to dress as she pleases. Flaunting her Mae West figure, Evelyn looks more like Miss Mona in "Best Little Whorehouse in Texas" than a broker. Her flamboyant and provocative style, however, shocks those who meet her. And she's often the target of unwanted come-ons. But she believes she's earned her right to, "show that I'm a woman as well as one hell of a salesman."

Woody Hochswender described this sexy, superfemale power dressing in *Vogue* as "aggressive, wildly exaggerated femininity—the controlling image is one of strength, even intimidation." But the woman who chooses such a tough but feminine, sexy but authoritative look can't rely on other people interpreting it as a power look. As the article warns, when "the wolf starts to howl, she had better be able to backchat like Madonna."

Then again, when you make yourself appear childlike and sexy as does Barbara, you *will* be taken seriously as a sex object, but you may not be taken seriously for much else by either men *or* women because the look bespeaks of inexperience, flakiness, lack of ability, and lack of purpose. In the wonderfully funny movie, *Working Girl,* secretary Tess McGill metamorphoses into a sleek Wall Street wheeler-dealer. As her long tresses hit the floor in favor of a more businesslike coif she correctly quips, "If you want to be taken seriously, you need serious hair."

Myth Two ⁓ *Youthful, physical attractiveness is the most important asset in the dating and marriage arena.*
If we believe what we see in magazines, TV, and movies, we'll come away

thinking that the average-looking adult woman just doesn't stand a chance with men. Youthful female sexuality shrieks at us from every newsstand and movie poster. *Cosmopolitan,* the monthly meeting of young beauty and sex, remains the most popular magazine of young adult women—the age when we establish the beliefs about our sexuality that we live with for the rest of our lives unless we challenge them somewhere along the way. But do the links between appearance and sex that saturate the media really set the standards for our individual sex lives?

To answer the question, I did a little sleuthing. The personals column in the *Los Angeles Times* offered the perfect post from which to watch men and women looking for a relationship. What better place to observe who wants what than in the home of Tinsel Town, where the media images we're bombarded with are bred and born?

ATTRACTIVE, LONG-LEGGED SBF [single black female], 38, with varied interests, seeks honest, tall SBM, 30+.

So read the first of more than 1,500 ads I combed through, searching for what women and men advertised about themselves and what they sought in a date. I looked at what each advertiser listed first, assuming that whatever he or she listed up front was most important. Then I checked further to see if physical appearance was mentioned somewhere else in each ad.

To no surprise, the women's ads emphasized their appearance. Forty-three percent described some aspect of their physical appearance *first.* All-in-all, three-fourths of the women touted one, if not more, physical characteristics.

Were my eyes ever opened by the men's ads, however! Having been out of the dating market for nearly two decades, but having been subjected to the same media blitz of breathtakingly beautiful young women that we see every day, nothing prepared me for what I found. More than half the men didn't specify *any* aspect of their desired date's appearance at all. And only two of the 900-plus men's ads mentioned some aspect of the desired woman's appearance *first*. So while the media leads us to believe that men are more interested in our physical charms than anything else, this wasn't the case in the ads I surveyed.

However, my findings don't mean that we've misread men all these years, and that our appearance really isn't all that important to them. They're interested in how we look all right, but in a much different way than the media leads us to believe. The fact is, at the *personal* level we operate within a much broader framework than society's narrow stereotype of the beautiful, young woman and the highly accomplished older man. And although stereotyped attractiveness is at the top of the list of adolescents and immature men with *Hustler* mentalities, most adult men find physical appearance to be but one of many interesting traits in their sexual partners. And what they consider attractive varies widely.

So how do we develop a new sexual identity in light of our aging bodies? While I can't give a pat answer, I can offer an example that may be helpful.

My friend Joanne and her husband Gary bought a beach condo just about the same time that Joanne turned fifty and hit the emotional skids over her aging appearance. The condo sits on a beach near a volleyball net where several girls' teams work out. Of course, everyone teased Gary about the girls, and he kidded back that he planned to organize his own team.

One night Joanne asked Gary if he still thought she was attractive, and he lovingly reassured her that she was just right. "But," he added, "you can't be captain of my girls' volleyball team." Instead of collapsing in a heap of tears, Joanne burst out laughing. At that moment, everything fell into place for her.

Young girls *are* attractive. And men *are* going to look at them. In fact, we *all* look at them because they are so beautiful. But they're not the *only* standard of attractiveness. That our beauty is *different* doesn't negate our full, ripe, and knowing brand of sex appeal—it just means that we may no longer want to be on a public beach in a thong bathing suit playing volleyball.

Several summers ago, I did a watercolor of an arrangement of white roses. If you grow roses, you know that those at summer's end are far different from the paler, smaller ones that come up in early spring. I was struck by how those roses of late August abounded with layer upon layer of petals that even in their whiteness ranged from pink to violet to blue. Each rose was gravid with scent and splayed out to the size of a salad plate.

Yet, we who've lived through the horror of losing a husband or lover may not feel like full-bodied roses as we wend our way through the dating maze. And this is especially true if we've been left for a woman who's half our age; for let's face it, while most men merely look at younger women, some *do* touch—never growing past their adolescent desire for women who aren't sexually mature. All too often middle-aged women find themselves back on the dating market. And when they do, the youth-versus-age issue looms large.

Cathy was served divorce papers, became a first-time grandmother of twins, and turned fifty all in the same year. On her own again after a thirty-year marriage, she returned to the dating scene while trying to cope with menopause, a shift in status from mother to grandmother, and, as she describes it, "towing my Philippine heritage that believes unmarried women shouldn't."

An attractive woman with liquid brown eyes and an ample figure, Cathy was pleased when Jerry, a man a few years older than she whom she'd known professionally for several years, asked her to dinner. But the evening didn't turn out as she envisioned at all. Although Cathy planned to get to know Jerry better during dinner in hopes that in time they might become more than mere friends, he spent the entire evening bragging about his prowess with the "young gals."

Cathy admitted later that Jerry never indicated anything other than a friendly interest in her and that it was she who wanted more. Yet what hurt Cathy more than the loss of a prospective lover was Jerry's unwillingness to relate sexually to someone her age. While she knew that men sometimes prefer much younger women, she hadn't been put in the embarrassing position of having to defend herself against this seemingly unjust situation.

After a flood of hot tears and a long night's discussion about aging bodies and what it means to grow into the fullness of our years, Cathy agreed that in her heart-of-hearts she didn't want a man whose sexual development had been stifled back in his teens. Although it was a hard lesson, what a difference this shift in attitude now makes in Cathy's dating and sex life!

When and if we're ever in a situation such as Cathy's, we need to remember that there are fifty-year-old men who still tuck *Playboy* under their beds and hit on their twenty-year-old secretaries, just as there are fifty-year-old women like Barbara who never grow past their senior prom night. But we must not allow these men's adolescent opinions to make us feel that we are unworthy. We aren't! We're sexually attractive in the fullest sense, and plenty of men appreciate that.

Myth Three — *All men stereotype women as sex objects.*
Recently the floodgates that previously held back the dirty secrets of incest, date rape, and child molestation have been thrown open. Sexual harassment, too, has had its share of the spotlight. As a result, we've reckoned with a world of men who sexually abuse women. In our catharsis, however, we may have failed to recognize that although some men treat women as mere sex objects, many don't.

We who teach know that an example of how *not* to do something won't show a student *how* to do it. So if we believe that most men view women primarily as sex objects, we're wise to rerecord that tape in our head by looking to those men who view us otherwise as models for change.

Despite the degree of sexual abuse or sexism we've experienced we can recall men who respected us for who and what we are capable of outside the boudoir. Male relatives, teachers, and neighbors often encourage young women to develop their talents. So do men coworkers and friends who see us sans the jaundiced eye of misogyny.

Even if you can name only a handful, spend some time thinking about how you feel when you're around men who empower you. Use the good feelings these men instill as a litmus test for your relationships with all men. The feelings of strength and ability they engender are what you are *entitled* as a woman to feel, because any man who makes you feel anything but positive about yourself toys with your fullness.

I believe that more men than we might recognize at first are aware of who we are and what we're capable of doing. When I sat down and thought about the men in my life, I realized that most men with whom I've worked respected me. In turn, working with these men strengthened my self-esteem and abilities, as well as my respect for them.

When it comes to our personal relationships, many men encourage their wives and significant others to explore, expand, and move beyond their sexual natures. This is certainly true in my marriage as well as in my parents' marriage. And I see the pattern repeated with my friends and their spouses or lovers. Rather than lock women into stereotyped sex roles, mature men want mature women in all their diverse fullness.

This was brought home to me as I sat at breakfast one warm fall morning and listened to Erica's story. Her clear blue eyes teared over periodically, but she kept talking until it all came out.

Erica's father sexually abused her, so she grew up never thinking of herself as anything more than an attractive body for men to look at and use. Not surprisingly, at eighteen she married Bill, a man much like her father. Though Bill pampered her with all the good things money could buy, he gave her no room to be anything other than his toy. Unbeknownst to Erica until years later, Bill sexually abused their beautiful daughter, Jenny, while she was in grade school.

After eighteen years of marriage, Erica begin to feel stirrings that "I was much more than just a sexy appearance." For six years Erica allowed that stirring to bubble up and prepare her for the inevitable divorce. "Then," she sighed, "I spent the next four years trying to put myself back together. I dug in deep and learned who I really was and what I could do."

Who was the *real* Erica? As she told me that morning, "I went in and found that the little girl who had been with me all along was talented and eager and ready to develop into a beautiful woman. I trusted her, and I followed her."

Truly, Erica is beautiful and powerful. She radiates. And she brims with fire to accomplish her life's work: Conducting workshops for victims of sex abuse.

Oh, by the way. Three years ago, Erica married David, a man who's as proud and supportive as he can be of his energetic, growing, giving wife.

Bowl Three: Parlor Power

The third bowl of lentils concerns our wounded belief that power comes from competing with other women in the appearance arena. But before we start on the bowl, I want to make it very clear that the wounded father's parlor is *not* the private domain of the rich and famous. Quite the contrary. Although it certainly is at home at the Beverly Wilshire and the Waldorf Astoria, the charity auction stare and all it represents are just as at home in bowling alleys on the south side of Chicago and at church suppers in Peoria and Ocala and Ft. Worth. For the drive to position ourselves in a hierarchy knows no monetary or geographic boundaries.

What having money *will* do is buy us more time to stay on the see-saw. This isn't a statement against money. Money is an inanimate object that is neither good nor bad. And personally, I *like* money. It's important to me to have money to buy the things I need and want. What I'm saying is that we can misuse it as we begin to see ourselves age. Like the emperor, we may continue to amuse ourselves with all the short-lived highs that come from dressing up for the parades rather than go into the kitchen and sift lentils.

So, when it comes to garnering the father's brand of power, it's not what we spend but how we *use* our appearance to control others. For example, some women maintain an antistatus position and disdain those who choose to follow fashion, treating them as if they don't have much to offer. Others armor themselves in powerful business attire and regard those who want to look sexy as incompetent. Let's remember that from our soul's perspective, each of these are examples of inauthentic uses of appearance.

To grow past this divisive use of our appearance, let's take our cue from Yellow, the caterpillar heroine in *Hope for the Flowers,* who began to feel that something was wrong with all the climbing. She left the heap, spun a cocoon, and turned into a beautiful butterfly who flew over the writhing mound of caterpillars on her way to a new life. Now that we, like Yellow, have gone into ourselves by sitting at Mother's tree, we also have the ability to rise above our old notions of what constitutes personal power.

To help us grow our butterfly wings, let's ask ourselves a question: What has a power-based appearance won for me?

This is a difficult question, for it demands that we analyze the way we look at our appearance and personal worth on any number of levels. But with the help of our inner wisewoman, we can determine honestly whether we or anyone else has gained from the expenditures of time, energy, money, and attention needed to maintain a wounded-power appearance. Too, it forces us to face the unpleasant truth that we may have lost more than we gained by playing the parlor game.

When I look back at when a status-based appearance was one of the major driving forces in my life, I see a lot of expended resources for which I gained practically nothing and had nothing to show for later. For example, what did looking better than anyone else at a professional meeting or party add to the long-term quality of my life? Not much, I must admit. Worse, I would have benefited *more* if I hadn't been so snared by the false parlor. I missed out on all kinds of chances to connect deeply with other people because I was so caught up in looking better than everyone else.

Unfortunately, the strangling effects of a hierarchical-based appearance far exceed the fact that we gain little from it. In truth, it puts us in a box that closes out the opportunities we must have if we want to move toward individuation.

As I discussed earlier, what we may feel we gain in personal power by armoring ourselves with the father's power isn't real power. It only gives us the illusion that we are mighty, and sooner or later the erroneous belief will bring us down.

Instead of letting us down, the power we found at the mother's grave is that of the loving and *inclusive* feminine, which enables us to rise higher and higher. It allows us to hear what our heart says, and then gives us the strength to carry it out. Her power gives us the sense of Self to say what must be said and to walk our own path. It allows us to warm up to the full possibilities in our lives, to other women who can have meaningful roles in our lives (absolutely irrespective of how they look), and to the ups and downs it takes to create a meaningful existence from our soul's perspective.

This isn't pie-in-the-sky-talk. It's *real*. Once we've determined to replace the wounded father's brand of power with our Mother's ancient potency, we can, for the first time, assess the power of our *authentic* appearance to help us fulfill those dreams and goals of our second half. What a gift! We have in us the same might as our foremothers, and, now that we've purified the appearance lentils, this potency is ours to use. Just as Denise realized that her size gives her a commanding platform from which to speak publicly about nutrition and Beverly claimed her mature good looks and physical presence as a big part of a personal power package that will assist her in a new career, we can do the same when it comes to accomplishing our soul's work.

And what of your soul's mission? Now that you've broken free of the parlor's hold on your appearance, tapped into the tree's sustenance, and purified the three bowls of lentils in the ashes, like Cinderella, you want to go to the festival—you want to get out into the world and *dance* to your inner tune.

My Appearance, My Life

Make a list of at least five major events in your life. Choose memorable times from your earliest childhood on. Leave enough space between them so that you can write a paragraph or two about each.

On a separate page, write down at least five major decisions you made during your life. Again, leave room for comments.

When you're finished, go back and reflect on each event and decision individually. Record any memories you have of how your appearance, clothing, grooming, personal image, or body played a role. You might recall the resources you spent, comments made to you about your appearance, feelings about your body that influenced your behavior in some way, others' expectations of or reactions to your appearance, or your reaction to other people's appearance. Also record any emotion that accompanies your memories, as well as any *shoulds* that surface.

Let your lists play on your mind for the next several days. Be open to what bubbles up. Like Denise and Beverly, you'll discover the role your appearance played in your development. This insight will lay the foundation for authentically empowering your appearance.

If Nature has prolonged our lives 25–40 years beyond menopause, it is vitally important to create/discover our purpose in the large picture, and to use our living, developing wisdom for the good of ourselves and those with whom we share life.

—Maura Kelsea, *Women of the 14th Moon*

⤙ Eight

Silver and Gold: Authentic Appearance

Cinderella gladly took the two bowls of clean lentils to her stepmother because she thought that she would be allowed to go to the festival. But the stepmother said, "These bowls will not help you. You have no clothes and you can't dance. We would be ashamed of you." So the stepmother turned around and hurried to the festival with her two daughters.

Left alone, Cinderella went to her mother's grave and wept, and she cried, "Shiver and quiver, little tree, silver and gold throw down over me."

And the bird threw down a gold and silver dress and slippers embroidered with silk and silver. She quickly put them on and went to the festival.

In true fairy tale style, the festival represents far more than a mere party. It's the time when the king's son will choose a wife from among all the maidens in the country. Since the king is the complete masculine, that makes his son the undeveloped masculine, just as Cinderella represents

159

the budding feminine. So rather than being just your run-of-the-mill ball, the festival symbolizes the place where a woman will be introduced to the masculine side of her psyche, what Jung called the *animus*.

Like Cinderella, we, too, have reached the stage in our quest for authenticity where we're ready to integrate our inner masculine energy. We've worked to expand our soul and cultivate the full feminine energy, and our soul hungers to be filled with the activating spirit that the animus brings us. For this is the only way we can bear the fruit that will fulfill the promise of our second half. In other words, we want to get out into what my students call the "real world" and do, by and for ourselves.

But Cinderella's stepmother never had any intention of letting her go to the festival. It's now clear that throwing more lentils into the ashes is a diversionary tactic. Her goal is for one of her own daughters, a maiden who's as cut off from the Great Mother as she, to marry the prince. Looking at it from this perspective, we realize that the last thing the dark side of our wounded feminine will allow us to do is integrate our ability to do outside of the confines of the parlor. She will accept nothing more or less than for us to remain entrapped in the appearance-based complex so that our stepsister ego can reign as queen of the parlor for the rest of our lives.

When you finally realize the truth that your ego has no intention of letting go of its hold on your appearance despite the work you do, you feel betrayed, just as Cinderella must feel. You've exposed every old belief regarding how you look. You've weighed alternatives and begun to develop the basis for making life-affirming choices when it comes to aging positively. Yet, it seems at this point like they're being thrown back in your face.

This inner war between ego and Self is to be expected, because we've only cleaned up our old, ego-based beliefs and behaviors—we haven't yet talked about the particulars of how you will look when you set out to dance with the enabling prince. From your ego's perspective, you attacked it and left it with nothing to attach itself to. And since it's the ego's job to create and maintain your public image, it's rightfully confused, fearful, and distraught.

Like Cinderella with the stepmother, you're in an in-between, or liminal, space. You're psychically and spiritually ready to move on, but your defensive ego simply won't let you. Since you don't yet know how everything is going to work out, your terrified ego demands that you turn around and go back to your old ways. A former president of my university called this the "Moses and the Israelites" syndrome. Even the slavery and fleshpots of Egypt begin to look pretty good when compared to wandering in the wilderness with a man who claims to talk to God through burning bushes and on fiery mountaintops.

Yet even though Cinderella is brokenhearted, she remains firm in her desire to go to the lifegiving festival. Although temporarily halted by the stepmother, she goes to her good mother's grave as she has so often before and weeps.

As the children of the true Mother, our desire to move forward in our individuation process now is stronger by far than our ego's demand that we stay seated near the parlor fireplace. Once a woman has come this far, Linda Leonard Schierse says that she "begins to sense the artificial quality inherent in the adoration of mere beauty or charm." So, rather than give in to the stepmother, we go to Mother and ask for silver and gold so that we can head for the festival and dance.

Authentic Beauty

Cinderella isn't the first character we've discussed who requested silver and gold. And she's not the first one who receives silk, either. The swindlers bilk the emperor out of his gold as well as yards and yards of silk yarn that they pocket. However, the spirit in which these precious materials are requested and the purposes for which they are used in the two stories are 180 degrees apart.

By asking for silver and gold, Cinderella indicates that the gray bed-gown and wooden clogs no longer serve her as they did while she lived the life of separation and introspection in the kitchen. She's saying that she's ready to be adorned in the beauty of light and life.

If you, too, have questioned up till now whether you might have to wear drab bedgowns for the rest of your life, take heart from Cinderella's request. We who have separated ourselves from the lure of the parlor have nothing to fear. Instead, we have every reason to rejoice, because we will soon wear beautiful dresses or scarlet fingernail polish or whatever else our heart desires.

I met Gayla, an aspiring artist, at the Jung Institute in San Francisco when I complimented a jasper ring she had on. Something about the ring seemed special, and my intuition was correct. Gayla told me that she had studied in a Buddhist monastery with a master who replaced the novices' secular clothing with nondescript shifts, claiming that they would be more attuned to their inner life if they were stripped of their former attire.

Gayla stayed with the teacher for three years, and then left to go on her own. Now she says, "I no longer even think about what's in fashion. Everything I put on is special. I've been given a gift—choosing my own clothing. And I'm not going to waste it." It was obvious that she bought the ring in that spirit.

Our Mother knows what a truly wonderful thing midlife beauty is, and she's never denied our desire to create a beautiful appearance. It's *we* who had to purify *our* parlor-contaminated concepts about beauty to the point that we no longer believe that our appearance is a standardized, commercial, youth-based commodity. Once we melt away the slag of those erroneous notions, however, we're ready to ask the Great Mother for authentic midlife beauty. And no sooner do we ask than she adorns us in splendor from head to toe.

To be sure, trying to define genuine beauty is difficult, for only the Great Mother knows its full scope. But throughout the centuries, one concept has been linked with beauty over and again: *truth*. Perhaps Keats said it best when he suggested that beauty is truth and truth is beauty. Yet to link beauty with truth in some esoteric way still leaves us way short of understanding the nature of the physical loveliness we desire, much less how to attain it.

But, if we keep the notion of truth in mind and connect it with Plato's belief that, "when a beautiful soul harmonizes with a beautiful form, and the two are cast in one mold, that will be the fairest of sights to him who has the eye to contemplate the vision," we begin to understand the nature of spirit-based beauty. And indeed, when Cinderella calls to the tree and asks for gold and silver, she is given the raw materials by which to develop her authentic appearance.

In Native American tradition, gold is the color of the ancient avatars who speak the truth as they guide us toward ever-higher planes. In the earliest Indo-Asian, Egyptian, European, and South American cultures, gold symbolized the sun—the highest and most potent masculine deity. It embodied power and accomplishment as well as truth, honor, and valor. So, as opposed to being sullied with the tricksters' wounded-masculine greed, the gold in Cinderella's dress adorns her in the ability to accomplish, energy, truth, honor, and love of the soul. In this, it foretells of her upcoming meeting with the enabling prince.

The silver in Cinderella's dress and shoes, of course, bespeaks of the moon and Cinderella's connectedness to the inner life of the kitchen and the ancient wisdom of the hazel tree. Silver imparts the complexity and multiplicity of the moon's phases, from the darkest dark to full-faced luminosity.

It's important that Cinderella's shoes, her means of getting where she is going, are made of silver and silk. Silk, remember, symbolizes the primal umbilical cord that connects earth with the sky and us with the Goddess. At this stage, although our goal is to meet the inner prince, like Cinderella, we're still under the primary protection and influence of the feminine.

If we look through the many versions of Cinderella's story, various accounts of what her dress is made of offer additional rich symbolism. One version has Cinderella dressed in sky blue, another in deep sea-green. In a third, she's given a dress as black as night. Others hold that her dress is as silver as the moon or as bright as the stars. Each of these variations conjures up imagery associated with the Great Mother and reaffirms Cinderella's quest for life, for her shining raiment symbolizes the ultimate triumph of the good mother over the dark stepmother.

Like Cinderella, when we make our desire for authentic beauty known, the white bird will dress us in a splendor that we never imagined before. Our only task is to open our hearts up to our intuition's wise council, to open our eyes to the vast possibilities, and to make our choices accordingly.

Our bodies and their adornment are as numinous today as were our earliest foremothers. If you want proof, consider trading clothes with someone for a while. Most of us wouldn't do it. Or at least we wouldn't trade with just anyone, because once someone has worn a garment, it becomes part of who she is—part of her persona as well as her aura. So when we put on her clothing, it's as if we put *her* on along with it. That's why teenagers are such notorious closet raiders. They're trying on various identities.

We don't have to trade clothes with someone to experience this. Unconsciously we attempt to take on another's essence when we try to look like a friend, mentor, or movie star. It's not merely the look we're after—the blond hair or the chic polish, it's a way of *being* her. We try to claim her charm or ability by draping ourselves in her look.

Although it may seem unrealistic that our bodies and adornment are still symbols of personal potential, given what we know of the past six thousand years that culminated in standardized fashion, it isn't at all. Indeed we retain our ancient power; it's just that the potency society assigned to how we look has worked against us instead of for us. So, time is nigh for us to regain and use our appearance power, for that's a big part of positive aging.

Radiant Beauty

By now it's obvious that genuine beauty has little to do with fashion or age and much more to do with aligning our appearance with our Self. When we dress from our hearts, as does Gayla, we dress in truth—because truth comes straight from the Self. When we dress in our own truth, as the Native Americans say, we walk in beauty. And funny thing, when we dress in the beauty of our Self, we appear more beautiful both to ourselves and others than we could ever have imagined, regardless of our wrinkles, sags, bags, or cellulite. It's as if a fairy godmother really does come down and touch us with her magic wand and make us into incredibly exquisite beings.

It's true. We see this in older women who dress from the heart. They radiate like Cinderella's dress and slippers, regardless of what they have on or how much money they spend. Their inner light is so strong that they exude a warmth and sheen that is beyond description. Such women are described by those who know them as being beautiful. And are people ever attracted to them!

To be sure, this brand of radiant mature beauty isn't the spring-green of our daughters or granddaughters, because it comes from having lived a good long while—having failed, survived, and prevailed—all the while being guided by the inner awareness that comes from the midlife quest. Also, when we say that Georgia O'Keefe or Jessica Tandy was beautiful, we're not talking merely about a physical look. We're echoing what news-woman Charlayne Hunter-Gault described in Cathleen Rountree's *On Women Turning 50,* when she said, "I have very concrete models in my life of women who have aged beautifully, creatively, energetically, and pro-ductively."

Mature women who have felt their inner call to shed their parlor-based image and go to the festival are like the silver moon—luminous and multifaceted. The women that come to my mind who fit this image, such as my mother, appear physically multidimensional—like they have several layers. Whereas women who've failed to plumb their depths appear rather flat and dull, regardless of what they have on or how many times they've had their faces peeled—you just can't get the patina of the moon from a jar of fruit acid.

This is because such women are powerful in the positive, Self-affirming sense of the word. Their potency comes from having welded their potential with accomplishment, their inner creativity with doing and being. Thus, their beauty wells up from *authentic* self-worth. This same determination to accomplish *our* life's mission, along with the genuine love we have in our hearts for ourselves and others, makes us radiant, too.

The key word, of course, is *love*. Before we can dress ourselves in the colors and textures of our souls, we must learn to love each and every part of our bodies. Then, when we are at the point where we really *adore* our physical self, we can *adorn* it in Spirit. It shouldn't be too big a surprise to learn that these two words have the same root meaning: *Praise*.

Body Love

Most of us have spent a lifetime trying to make ourselves attractive without seeing just how beautiful we really are. I'm not talking about recognizing how good we look after getting a new haircut. I'm talking about being aware that our bodies truly are beautiful temples of our glorious Selves. Since such common gratitude is so often missing, it's time we become aware of and grateful for how incredible they are.

The best way to learn to love your body is to take one part at a time and give it some love—look at it, think of how it has helped you over the past decades, and then thank it for being there for you all these years. As you're comfortable, work through all parts of your body. You might want to pick a different part each day and stay with it a while. Start with those that haven't caused you problems or attracted negative attention from others. Save those parts for when you are ready. But don't neglect them. Even your bulging thighs are part of your beautiful body. It may take some time to learn to love and appreciate them, but you will.

I often look down at my hands while I'm writing. I like their shape and color as well as what they've done for me. They've watercolored, and they've gotten splinters from renovating too many old houses. They're scarred here and there from kitten claws and puppy teeth. They type my words and rub cream on me. Mine are not the hands of a child. They're the hands of a middle-aged woman, wrinkled and worn like well-used kid gloves.

Learning to love each part of our body doesn't have to be all that serious, either. In *Revolution from Within,* Gloria Steinem described the age spots on her hands as having a sense of humor. Similarly, Elaine, a woman in her mid-forties who participated in one of my seminars, chaffed a bit as she tried to think of something to love about her ample hips. After a few minutes she said in all good fun, "Well, they keep me from having to take a padded stadium seat to my son's soccer games." It's time we all took our cues from these two wise women and lighten up on our bodies.

As we do so, we free ourselves to expect less than fashion-photo perfection from our bodies. What a payoff this is! Since no body is picture-perfect anyway, when we learn to love ours because of how perfectly functional it is and what a gift it is, we relieve stress from our bodies. Yet, if relieving stress weren't enough of a boon itself, praising our bodies helps them to look and perform even better.

As you recognize the incredible value of each part of your body, you begin to ask yourself questions like, "How could I cut off pieces of or want to completely change this good friend who has given me so much and is so uniquely mine? Why would I want my nose or breasts to look just like everyone else's? By whose authority is it that the only acceptable skin is wrinkle free?"

Through answering such questions from the perspective of your Self, you come to view your body not only as a gift but as a responsibility. Since we were raised believing that our bodies belonged to anyone and everyone but us, this is a major feat. But once you've taken dominion over it, you begin to go out of your way to treat your body like a loved one.

What do you do for those whom you love and who have entrusted you with the power to care for them? You tend their needs, speak kindly of them, protect them from harm, position them in the best light possible, and give them gifts. To be sure, these are the same activities that make up the whole notion of adorning our bodies in a way that enhances authentic appearance.

Sensing True Worth

Once we've learned to love our bodies, we can begin to reconnect them to our Selves. Just as we reunited with the essence of the good mother through the sights, sounds, smells, feels, and tastes of nature, we now can use our sensory arsenal to bridge the severed lifeline between our inner and outer.

Let's start with the positive uses of scent. American society has turned its collective nose up at the idea of natural body odors to the point that any natural scent is offensive. Yet, while anthropologists argue that this is a loss of no small magnitude, as individual women, we're in no position to break with tradition lest we be ostracized. But social convention doesn't preclude us from enjoying our own body scents in the privacy of our own sanctuaries. We've been programmed to think of ourselves as sweet-smelling little girls and anything more odiferous as evil. Yet, we are viable, juicy women who smell of Mother's musty earth.

Most of us never discovered our unique scents, because we're too busy covering them up with commercial ones. Unfortunately, however, research shows that women buy perfume because of name and product image, rather than scent. This is a wholesale waste of money! To buy Joy simply because it is the most expensive perfume on the market or Chanel Nº 5 because of its sophisticated image shoves body and soul further apart.

The ancients knew that scent is powerful, and they were careful with the essences they used. We, too, say a lot about ourselves when we apply a fragrance. So it's up to us to choose how we *want* to smell. What does your perfume say about you? What does it say *to* you? By all means, avoid those pseudo-psychological tests in magazine articles that correlate personality characteristics with various well-known brands. Scent is far too personal to be standardized like that.

In addition to wearing scents that are really *you,* wash your surroundings in a carefully selected scent. Using candles, incense, potpourri, and bowls of scented water to help us accomplish everything from getting over the flu to going into deep meditation is as old as humankind, so you don't need an aromatherapist to help you learn the value and use of scent. Your body already knows what it needs and likes, and your best tactic is to take yourself to a good candle or herb shop and put your nose to work doing what it does best.

Once you've invested in some personally meaningful scents, really *use* them to connect with your Self. If you light a candle when you bathe, take a moment and breathe in the scent and imagine it going all over your body and relaxing each muscle. Close your eyes and envision the scent's color and texture. Is it as satiny-smooth as purple silk or like starched, crisp cotton? Burn sage or incense as part of your prayers or meditation and inhale the aroma. Visualize it moving into each part of your body and dematerializing the day's grime. Then move the evocative scent into your Self. What a way to open up your body and soul to your higher being! Remember, the concept that your body has a metaphysical quality is no oxymoron. Everything in the universe is made of energy—it's just that our bodies are dense, whereas spirit isn't.

In addition to reconnecting to our bodies through scent, we need to get to know them through touch. As you rub on cream, concentrate on how it feels to your thigh and hip. Love your arms, legs, and neck as you would love a pet by rubbing and patting it. Words cannot describe the intense message you send your body through the warmth of your hand when you practice this on a daily basis. As you stroke your body get to know every freckle and wrinkle. This is not a sin; it's your body.

Keep in mind that those parts of your body you have the hardest time touching need the most love, for they are the ones you've disenfranchised over the years through negative thinking. So give them extra attention.

As you caress your body, do so with no strings attached. Your body serves you just as it was made to serve. When it comes to loving your face, sagging breasts, or hips, take your cue from the good Mother who attaches no strings to you because she accepts you just the way you are.

Just as you become aware of how your body feels to your hand, also become aware of how your clothing and makeup feel on your body. Experience how blusher brushes tickle your skin. What do various fabrics you wear feel like? Does your body enjoy wearing them or not?

Texture is probably the most overlooked stimuli in our perceptual field. Yet, when it comes to really living in our bodies, texture is so important, because it keeps us grounded in the physical moment. We were given bodies for good reason—so that we can live in the physical world rather than float off into spirit. When we take a moment to experience the textures we have on, we're brought back to our physical reality from out of daydreams, the work we've gotten caught up in, or whatever our mind is busy thinking about. Thus we stay tuned to what's going on around us—to what's going on in life right here and *now*.

Feel your jewelry as you wear it. Is it heavy against your skin or light as a feather? Cool or warm? Believe it or not, how your jewelry feels against your body makes a difference in how you think and act. When you become aware of the way you react to the various textures, weights, and feel of metals and other materials, you begin to make choices as to the statement you want to make to others as well as what you want to accomplish each day.

Although we may be unaware of it, the sound our clothes make has just as much impact as how they look and feel. Each sound differs in quality and meaning. If you haven't listened to your clothes and jewelry lately, give it a try. You may be surprised at what you're saying about yourself each morning when you get dressed.

Silent clothes and shoes allow us to stay to ourselves. At the other end of the spectrum, women who want to be noticed are loud in color and style as well as voice. We can hear them. Sometimes we even say that their appearance is brassy, because their jewelry jingle-jangles, their heels click, and their slips rustle.

Taste may at first appear difficult to incorporate into our appearance unless we're into edible underwear or chewing on our blouse collars like a second-grader. But taste is valuable, and we shouldn't ignore it. When it comes to scents, colors, and sounds, we say that we can almost taste them. And it's true. Our mind assigns a certain taste to them, because taste is part of our overall metaphysical sensory package. This explains why so many interior and fashion colors have edible names such as cream, cantaloupe, sage, and cherry. Seeing these rich colors makes our mouth water.

On the biophysical level, we who honor our bodies learn to relish the taste of those foods that nourish them best. Juicy berries and other fruits, crystal pure water, nutty-flavored whole grains, and leafy green vegetables are our bodies' life sources. Eating these foods in abundance while retraining our taste buds to get over their craving for meat, saturated fats, refined sugars, and alcohol will do more to make us beautiful (both inside and out) than all the cosmetics and plastic surgery that money can buy.

The Eye of the Beholder

I've purposefully saved sight until last, because it's the sense that we can relate to our appearance the easiest, and the visual field is where all our other senses come together to form our personal image. So, until we've developed an appreciation for how we can enhance our bodies and reconnect them to our Self via scent, touch, sound, and taste, a discussion of sight is premature.

Once we grow to love our bodies through the other four senses, we automatically love what we see on both the metaphysical and physical planes. Gone are the days when we judge our appearance by how it visually measures up to two-dimensional photos in magazines and three-dimensional other women, because, as we came to our senses by using them to get to know and love our physical selves, we also came to know, understand, and appreciate our God-given individuality. And, as soon as we love our bodies' uniquenesses, we never again think of them as ugly or inferior.

This doesn't necessarily mean that we will dismiss all standards of female beauty we previously judged ourselves against, at least not until there are formidable enough numbers of us to create social change. Even then there will still be standards. They'll just be broader in scope.

However, as we learn to cherish our individual appearance, we begin to put society's standards of female beauty into perspective. Just as there are standards against which we judge beauty in any visual art form, be it painting or sculpting, certain desirable characteristics in the female anatomy will prevail when it comes to cultural taste. It is inevitable that certain women will *naturally* come closer to this standard than others. Truly, some women have bone structures and body proportions that seem to have been fashioned by Aphrodite herself.

As we link body to Self, we retrain our eyes to view that type of rare female beauty as a gift, just as having a beautiful voice or talent for turning a phrase are gifts. But this special kind of beauty won't serve as the standard by which we're all judged and for which we all strive. So, when we look upon a Catherine Deneuve or Grace Kelly, we won't castigate ourselves. Rather, we'll enjoy her beauty and be pleased for her that she has it—no more, no less.

Claiming Our Fullness

As you realign your perception of your body, you begin the process of reclaiming the ancient feminine in the full sense of the word. For centuries now women have been stereotyped as being passive rather than active—as receivers rather than doers. Cinderella's stepmother chides her and tells her that she can't dance and therefore has no business going to the festival—virtually the same message we've received all our lives in one form or another. But now that we understand what all our bodies do, we realize that there's nothing passive about the mechanics of the female body.

It isn't hard then to take the next step of loving the *look* our bodies acquire as they go about their business of doing. For truly, if our bodies *do,* they're going to get a little worn around the edges. Our wrinkles and our rough hands attest to the fact that we are capable doers and have been for some time. One of my favorite quips regarding the empowered look of the older woman comes from Cathleen Rountree's *On Women Turning 50,* when activist-lawyer Gloria Allred says, "If and when I develop more wrinkles than I have now, I'll wear them as medals of survival and not be concerned about them."

Silver and Gold

Now that we understand the nature of positive aging, it's time to shake the tree and ask the good Mother for silver and gold. As we do, we realize that adorning ourselves in socially dictated clothing is no longer our goal. To expect that we could merely go back to dressing ourselves for the same reasons that we did formerly would be a return to the parlor mentality. No, the new splendor of silver and gold is something much more.

I cannot say what is in store for each of you as you mine your depths for the Mother's gifts. I can say for certain, however, that a unique and glorious drive was planted in you at birth, which now cries out to be tended. James Hollis put it this way in *The Middle Passage,* "Finding and following our passion, that which touches us so deeply that it both hurts and feels right, serves individuation by pulling our potential from the depths."

So the power of the Mother within us is to recognize our dreams and hearts' desires. In addition to creativity, Her arsenal includes the power of infinite and authentic emotion—of feeling joy and sadness in their full spectrum from each layer of our being. It is the strength to believe that which comes from our inner Self wholeheartedly, without shame or apology. It is the power of love—selfless, all encompassing, compassionate, and unqualified. Finally, it's the strength to stand on our convictions, sans the stepmother's fear.

In wearing the Mother's silver and gold you incarnate her power in your appearance so that you can operate in the physical world, just as Cinderella is fortified when she wears them to the festival. Since your divine Self dwells deep within you, you bring its essence to the surface by wearing jewelry or colors or other symbols of all that is positive within you. In this way, wearing a sacred symbol works like a pump that continuously bathes your psyche in the magical waters of your Self. You've done this all along if you wear a cross or a Star of David as the symbol of your religious beliefs. The insignia gives you something concrete to wear on the outside that stands for internal beliefs, which are otherwise difficult to conceive. Thomas Merton writes that such a symbol, "contains in itself a structure which awakens our consciousness to a new awareness of the inner meaning of life and of reality itself." So, when we adorn ourselves in symbols of the Mother, Her essence is brought up from our deepest parts and empowers us.

While it's true for the most part that we've lost the ancient connect-edness with spirit that was inherent in home-produced cosmetics, cloth-ing, and jewelry, there are ways to personalize our appearance in honor of our newly discovered Self and her desire to go to the festival. For to be sure, few of us want to or can return to the time when women wove cloth and scouted the countryside for berries with which to make dyes and makeup.

So guess who supplies the raw materials for a spirit-based appearance? None other than the tricksters themselves. The fruits of Seventh Avenue now are ours to pick and use as we wish with no strings attached. For, when we mined the treasure of the tree, we negated the trickster's power to keep us in the parlor in clothes that rob us of our birthright as beautiful daughters of the true Mother. To help you with this ironic yet awesome task, turn to the white bird in one of her many guises and ask for silver and gold so that you can go to the festival. Just as she came to Cinderella, she'll come to you via your inner child, wisewoman, or any one of her other manifestations.

The Magic Child

If you remember back to Denise's and Beverly's stories, both women expressed regret that they let either their own or someone else's narcissis-tic way of thinking stop them from carrying out a childhood dream. This is not uncommon. It happened to me more times than I care to recount, and my guess is that as you thought about your life's decisions it cropped up again and again. Yet despite its somber base there's a lesson here, and one that's going to be a barrel of fun.

Your inner child was wise long before she was lured into the parlor. She knew of your potential and life's purposes, and given full reign she'll direct you right to the doorstep of your heart's deepest desires. So, I sug-gest that you set your inner child loose at the mall and let her play dress up again. I'm serious. Take her to Lord and Taylor or Macy's or Kmart—wherever she wishes—and let her go. She still can teach you a thing or two about expressing yourself. Does she want some candy-colored lipstick? Fine, buy it for her. Maybe she prefers to have a football helmet. Get out your MasterCard™. Then put on that pink lipstick and go throw a football up in the air a few times. It's amazing what you might dream up to *do* next.

In actuality, you've done this all your life. You just didn't know who was calling the shots at the time. Remember the teal-green satin blouse that hangs in the closet because it doesn't match anything else and isn't your usual tailored style? Your inner child must have slipped into the store with you the day you bought it. If so, put it on, stuff it into a pair of jeans, and take that little girl for a walk in the park!

Sacred Color

It's also time to mine your true colors. If you keep a dream journal, go back through it and look for repeated references to specific colors. Start noticing colors that seem to "speak" to you as you go about your daily activities. You'll soon see that four or five colors appear more vibrant than the rest or resonate within you in an inexplicable way. These are your personal, sacred colors. Wear them and they'll open you up to spirit. You'll be surprised how good you feel in them, how good they look on you, and how other people respond to you when you wear them. Remember when you wear these special colors they resonate with your aura, and you *radiate*.

In addition to wearing your personal colors, claim the particular power of the colors in the medicine wheel, the chakras, or any other ancient color system wherein colors represent various manifestations of spirit. In almost every tradition, blue sings of water and air, and green smells of the earth. According to Native American tradition, turquoise reigns over the Southwest, the direction of dreams.

As I discussed earlier, the goddesses each have their own colors, and you align yourself with them by wearing their special hues. I mention goddesses on purpose, because at this juncture of your journey, the colors that link you to the feminine will serve you best, just as Cinderella's dress and shoes weigh heavier with silver than gold.

What I'm speaking of in general terms as being feminine are the colors that reflect the inner realm of intuition, emotion, dreams, and visions rather than the outer world of acting and doing. Although acting and doing are our ultimate goals, neither Cinderella nor we have met the prince yet. We're only just getting dressed so that we can go from the tree to the festival.

We in midlife transition especially need to incorporate the colors of the ancient wisewoman. Black bespeaks of Hecate and Grandmother Spider, and white of the northern Native American concept of grandmother wisdom. And it's no mere happenstance that elderwomen everywhere wear purple. In almost every ancient tradition violet transcends the physical plane and takes us straight into the realm of spirit.

Not only do the sacred colors, themselves, swell our soul in special ways, but so do their various shades. Dark and muddied shades such as navy, wine, and forest green resonate with the night, the dark moon, and the inner life, whereas brighter hues like emerald, royal, and ruby burst forth with active daylight, and light colors and white sing the song of angels.

Primary colors—red, blue, and yellow—are saturated with single potency. At their fullest, they're associated with childhood, for innocent children love their single, simple, yet powerful messages. Other colors, those that are blended from the primary colors, such as butter cream, seafoam, salmon, and aubergine, bespeak of complexity and multidimensionality. So, choose your colors well and wear them wisely. Since they are pregnant with symbolism, they command your respect and attention.

Line and Design

The styles of clothing you choose are as symbolic as the colors you wear. So it's up to you to dip your cup into Mother's mighty river and drink from it as you dress each morning. In choosing styles, motifs, fabrics, and textures you might look to your roots. Ethnic clothing became popular in the sixties, when we first began to question society's penchant for soulless fashions. Our desire for clothing that was close to the earth and the old ways as we transcended from child to maiden stemmed directly from our need to reconnect with our roots.

As we transition into yet another phase in our life cycle, it's important to garner the power and abilities of our mighty heritage both as individuals and as women in general. The first layer of my soul lives in the black dirt of northwest Texas and the rolling hills north of Austin. This is my homeland, for it is the country of my grandmothers and great-grandmothers—Texas women who pioneered the wilderness with the strength of an army. Although I was raised in a city far later than the days when they crossed rivers and plains in rickety wagons and watched helplessly as their babies died of unnamed summer fevers, when I shut my eyes and feel these women in my bones, I'm filled with their determination not merely to survive but to prevail. And when I don boots and long flounced skirts I'm no drugstore cowgirl; I do so in reverence to the legacy of their iron-clad spirits.

Because we are all of one ancient bloodline, the desire to reconnect to distant heritages also resides within us, and so we may nourish ourselves by wearing their symbols. And while there is no better way to redeem and honor our connectedness with all women than by adorning ourselves in each other's symbolic clothing, a word of caution is in order. The fashion industry routinely puts ethnic-inspired costumes on the runways, thereby reducing them to mass produced products that are bereft of their original spirit. Look-a-like Navajo jewelry is produced in factories in Taiwan. And you can buy "Indian Madras" blouses that are factory dyed in Jamaica with synthetic colors that are guaranteed not to bleed.

I recently found a pair of exquisite brass and copper earrings at an art show at the Los Angeles County Museum that had what appeared to be an African woman tooled onto a flat shield-shaped background. I was intrigued and would have purchased them until I asked the man at the booth to tell me about them. He had no idea who the woman was. After I probed a bit, he reluctantly told me that the earrings were mass produced here in the United States. I shook my head and walked on.

Indigenous groups resent this piracy, and I don't blame them one bit. So, I don't advocate that we wholesalely adopt other peoples' ethnic costumes and jewelry as our own *unless* we do it in the name of the same spirit for which the items were originally created. In this way, we honor both the holy garments and the people who first deemed them sacred.

Just Rewards

The cultural tenet that women don't *do* and simply *are* is ridiculous. Of course we *do*. We've been doing all our lives. We've developed careers, had babies, cooked and sewn, learned, organized, raised money, planted gardens, and engaged in a thousand other activities. But despite all that we've accomplished, at some point in our lives most of us look back and grieve over the fact that we haven't *done* anything.

Why is it that we so often ignore all the dances we've attended and, instead, agree with the stepmother that we can't and, therefore, shouldn't go to the festival that will propel us into the second half of our lives? It's because we've neither gotten credit for what we've done nor have allowed ourselves to take credit for having done it. To accept credit and the rewards of our labor wouldn't have been to the liking of either society or our low self-esteem. Our work, like our beauty, had to have been done for others—for the good of the family, so that somebody else could go to college, so that the boss or the department would look good, and so on. As a result, we worked and did and accomplished so anonymously that now our numerous achievements are invisible even to ourselves.

But it's time for all that to change. It's time for us to pat ourselves on the backs and thank ourselves for what we have done in our lives. Otherwise, how will we ever satisfy the innate urge to accomplish the mission of our upcoming decades?

There's no better way to congratulate ourselves for being the doers we are than through giving ourselves jewelry, for no aspect of our adornment is as symbolic. That society warped the primal symbolism of gold and silver into the wounded masculine symbols of economic clout doesn't negate their ability to impart the spirit of the Divine Feminine, but it does require that we understand just *how* to reward ourselves with it.

Regardless of how we acquire it, jewelry bears out the legacy from the days when the patriarchs of old asserted their dominion over women. Make no mistake, modern-day bracelets, necklaces, rings, ankle chains, and earrings still harbor back to the time when they were symbols of female bondage and male wealth. Even until quite recently, it just wouldn't do for a woman to buy fine jewelry for herself. It was considered vulgar and tasteless as well as a threat.

I remember being a freshman in college and buying myself a gold and topaz ring. My macho-jock boyfriend threw a fit and made me promise that I wouldn't tell anyone else who had bought it. The relationship didn't last but a couple of weeks after the incident, but I never forgot the shock I felt at his wrath and insecurity. His outburst didn't stop me from buying more jewelry, but it did bring home jewelry's tainted history as the symbol of female passiveness and male domination.

When it comes to adorning our bodies with precious metals and stones we, as individuals, can't change society's notions about who buys what for whom and what it symbolizes. But mass societal change isn't our aim here. Right now we're working on symbolically empowering *ourselves* to meet the decades and tasks ahead. So, even though we're the only one who knows what a pair of earrings or a bracelet stands for, when we buy it with money we either save up by sacrificing other things we want or by earning the money ourselves (gift money won't do here), it empowers us by helping us get past the notion that our worth must be bestowed on us by others—husbands, lovers, parents, or whomever.

This doesn't mean that we want to eschew gift jewelry altogether, for jewelry that's given to us by others has a power that can be quite positive. If, for instance, you gain your grandmother's strong determination by wearing a ring you inherit from her, so much the better. But we are *personally* strengthened to expand the potential of the fullness of our life, by and through ourselves, when we buy our own jewelry.

I really like wearing earrings. Other women are partial to bracelets or rings, but earrings really do something special for me. So, for years I've bought earrings to reward myself for accomplishing something I deem worthwhile. I bought gold loops when I went to Mexico to research women's appearance. When I gave research papers at conferences in Singapore and Istanbul I bought gold earrings. The day I finished the first draft of this book I bought more loops, and I bought the most beautiful pair of Navajo sterling and turquoise earrings with part of my first book advance.

These earrings make up part of my personal achievement package. And to be sure, when I wear them, I can feel the energy they impart. As need be, I put them on to give me strength, as expressions of joy, to get me through rough spots on my journey, and sometimes for no apparent reason other than I feel that I might need what a certain pair might have to offer that day.

So, too, I wear the earrings I've earned as expressions of thanksgiving for my talents and opportunities and in praise to God for bestowing life on me. Physically displaying my gratitude via their symbols, shapes, and colors, of course, results in being granted so much more of the same. For when we return the favor of life, either through symbolic prayers or by making something of our talents, we demonstrate on a metaphysical plane that we are worthy of our gifts. This is an especially important lesson for midlife women who are entering that time when honoring our highest creativity and abilities becomes paramount.

Dressing for the Festival

We know that Cinderella's dress and shoes are magnificent, so we, too, can expect to look radiant as we step up to dance with the prince. But the story gives us no hint as to exactly *what* it is that will make us glow. That's because each of us varies so greatly that we have a personal brand of beauty. So before we head for the festival, therefore, we must learn to adorn our individuality for the particular roles we play.

Indeed, like stage troopers who schlep costumes and grease-paint from one theater to the next, we put on appearances so that we, too, can act out our roles. Sociologist Erving Goffman calls the various looks we create "identity kits" because they align so closely with and help us perform our various parts.

Just as with actors, the more we *look* the part, the more effective we are to our audience. For example, on arriving home one evening Laura, a lawyer, expected a spirited greeting from her three-year-old grandson, Tim. But Tim barely looked up from his pint-sized trucks. Too tired to stop and ask questions, Laura went and changed into sweats. When she came back into the room where Tim played, he jumped up, ran to her, and squealed, "Grammy, *now* you're home." Same woman, same child, yet Laura's appearance made all the difference to Tim. From Tim's perspective, Laura *became* his grandmother when she put on her grammy clothes, because the approachable sweats indicated how they would spend the evening. Conversely, however, a judge and jury would say, "no way" if Laura showed up in court wearing the sweats that Tim preferred.

As with Laura, our clothing, makeup, jewelry, and hair styles not only identify our roles but also *legitimize* us as qualified to play them out—both to ourselves and to those with whom we interact. And, while it's true that all of us—men, women, children—dress for the parts we play, women who have danced with a wounded animus most of their lives often feel as though they costume themselves to play an alien role. In some strange, unexplainable way they perceive themselves as masked impostors who merely act out their role as teacher or nurse but are unconnected from their actions. Of course, these women feel this way because they *have* made themselves into impostors, masked players who cater to other people's *shoulds,* in order to keep their fragile egos afloat.

But we who have reconnected to our Self and developed authentic appearance no longer feel like we're pretending. Instead, we experience ourselves directly as *doers.* And does this ever pay off, both physically and psychically. Before working to remove her false parlor persona, Laura used her business attire to boost her confidence. She used her suit to say, "I am playing the part of a lawyer." Now when she puts on her suit and walks into the courtroom, however, every fiber of her being says "I *am* a lawyer."

The difference is that Laura now draws from her own power source, and she holds onto her power. She can do this because dressed both in her awareness of Self as well as her suit, she identifies with her abilities. She accepts *her* accomplishments and learns from *her* failures. Too, she speaks from her own authority, verbally and symbolically. Can't you just feel the difference between the old days when Laura put on a suit to give her self-confidence as opposed to now putting on a suit *because* of her confidence? The radiant energy that emanates from her can't be missed. As time goes by, she'll become even more effective in that her Self-accepting and Self-congratulatory attitude will spiral her up and up.

But, while Laura has gone to the festival and met her prince, we haven't. So the time has come for us to put on the colors and symbols of our powerful Self and wend our way from the tree to the castle.

Reward Time

Begin to purchase jewelry for yourself, and then wear it in tribute to who you are and what you have accomplished. It makes no difference whether it's a platinum pendant or a wrist chain of the tiniest silver links, because neither price nor size matters. And neither does quantity matter. This isn't a contest where amassing the most wins the biggest pot of Mother's power. What matters is that you purchase the silver and gold you need and wear it in honor of your *own* ability to *do*.

Allowing our true spirit to have the natural balance of the full range of our masculine and feminine within requires a shift in consciousness. When we allow our true spirit to manifest itself, we are acting on all that we know that lies within us. We cannot allow gender stereotyping to prevent us from becoming who we can be.

—Marilyn J. Mason, *Making Our Lives Our Own*

Nine

The Prince: Appearance Power

When Cinderella arrived at the festival, her stepsisters and stepmother didn't recognize her. She looked so beautiful they thought that she was a foreign princess.

When the prince saw Cinderella he would dance only with her. If anyone else asked her to dance, he said, "This is my partner."

Cinderella danced until evening, and then she wanted to go home. But the King's son said, "I will go with you and keep you company," for he wanted to see to whom the maiden belonged.

Cinderella escaped from him, however, by jumping into the pigeonhouse. The prince waited until Cinderella's father came by and told him that the strange maiden had leapt into his birdhouse.

The old man thought, "Can it be Cinderella?" He asked for a pickax and chopped the pigeonhouse to pieces. But no one was in it, for Cinderella had jumped down from the back of the pigeonhouse, run to the hazel tree, and taken

*off her beautiful clothes and laid them on the grave so that the bird could take
them back.*

*When the family got home, they found Cinderella asleep in the ashes in her
dirty gray bedgown. A dim oil lamp burned on the mantle near her.*

*The next day when everyone had gone, Cinderella went once more to the tree
and asked for silver and gold to be thrown down to her. Then the bird threw down an
even more beautiful dress. And when Cinderella arrived at the festival, everyone was
astonished at her beauty.*

*The king's son had waited for her and danced only with her until evening came
and Cinderella wanted to leave. Yet again, the prince followed Cinderella home. But
she ran into the garden and scampered up a beautiful pear tree, scurrying like a
squirrel, until the prince lost sight of her.*

*As before, the prince waited and told the father that the maiden had climbed
into the tree. And the father thought, "Can it be Cinderella?" Whereupon he asked for
an axe and cut down the tree, but no one was in it. When the family returned,
Cinderella again lay among the ashes.*

*On the third day, Cinderella once more went to the hazel tree, and the bird
threw down the most magnificent dress yet. And the slippers were pure gold. She
looked so beautiful that no one at the festival could speak.*

*Again the prince danced only with Cinderella and told those who approached,
"This is my partner."*

*When evening came, Cinderella escaped so fast that the prince couldn't follow
her. But he had the staircase smeared with pitch, which stuck to Cinderella's left
slipper when she ran down to leave.*

The prince picked it up, and it was small and golden.

Cinderella's experiences during the three day festival are so rich in
symbolism, wisdom, and instruction that an entire book could be written
on them alone. For the festival and the activities swirling around it are the
story of the initial meetings between the feminine and the masculine. As
discussed in the last chapter, integrating our inner masculine is the final

part of our quest for authentic appearance. In this, it opens the way for us to activate our midlife potential.

Major motion pictures that portray strong and capable women, such as *Out of Africa,* and TV series like "Dr. Quinn Medicine Woman" often spawn clothing styles that attest to our deep-seeded desire to weld talent with action. To be sure, "Murder She Wrote" probably did more to establish a chic, can-do image for the over-fifty-five woman than the now defunct *Lear's* magazine ever could have, because Jessica Fletcher *acted* on her own initiative and intuition rather than merely being an inanimate image. However, celluloid role models will bear fruit only if we wear their self-activating image to the festival and meet our animus.

As the animus has everything to do with how we live in the physical world, failing to dance with him leaves women in what I call the "soap opera" or "torch novel" syndrome. Most of us enjoy a good bodice-ripper novel now and then, and there's nothing quite like *An Affair to Remember* to set our hearts stirring. But women who fail to meet the prince become numbed to their *own* potential. Unable to energize their authentic feelings, desires, and abilities into action, they let others' lives vicariously fill them with a pseudolife and can end up *entrapped* in other's lives—their children's, husband's, neighbor's, or favorite TV character's.

As Marie-Louise von Franz writes, "When women have an undeveloped animus, when they have not worked on the animus, their mental functions often remain fixed on gossip and thinking about their neighbors." To be sure, this unfortunate state has nothing to do with whether women are stay-at-home wives or business tycoons. It has to do with our not taking our turn on the dance floor and thereby not vivifying our inner voice and giving it a chance to sing in public.

Given that failing to go to the festival will swamp us with the stagnation, helplessness, and hopelessness that turns us into gossip-mongers and control freaks, we might wonder why more women don't get out and take a whirl around the floor with the prince. The answer is simple. Going to the festival and meeting the prince is no ball. In fact, it's the biggest hurdle we face as we move through our middle passage. It took Cinderella the magic three attempts, and it may take us as many months or years.

The King's Invitation

Since the Disney version has Cinderella falling into the arms of the prince at a royal ball that ends at midnight, you may be surprised that the festival in the earlier version is a daytime affair. This is because Cinderella goes to the festival of the good king, the archetype of the complete masculine, on his turf and in the full light of his symbolic sun. And it's this mandate that we must move into the realm of the masculine in order to meet the prince that terrifies some women.

The very patriarchy who raised human kings to gods buried the archetypal Good King as surely as it did away with the good mother, leaving us not only with a wounded masculine society but with a nagging, perfectionistic, competitive, wounded animus who jabs at us in our daylight hours and haunts our dreams at night. This is why many women recoil in dread before male gods, even as they worship them, and others opt to turn their backs on traditional religious tenets altogether.

It's not just wounded tenets that leave women loathe to develop their masculine sides, it's that most of us have been dancing with one part of our wounded animus or another all our lives. In an attempt to break down gender barriers, some of us emulated our dads or identified with the collective masculine, patterning our attitudes and ways of doing after them, while eschewing the feminine. But by the late '80s we who took our fathers to our first dance began to realize that instead of accomplishing great things, we were still dancing—harder and faster than ever. And for all our fancy footwork, we were as bereft of personal meaning as society itself. Others of us tried to complete ourselves by marrying a man (or men) who seemed to possess the qualities we thought we lacked in ourselves—power, experience, status, and the ability to generate wealth. But too many of us ended up as disillusioned as the fathers' daughters, for other people's power and status too easily oppress and entrap us, leaving us depleted and unfulfilled.

So, we who've sat under the peaceful tree of the good mother are rightfully skeptical of going out on another date. Despite our misgivings, however, one day the king issues forth an invitation for us to come meet the prince—to reclaim the hero/god in us.

When I received the invitation, I trembled at having to go dance with the masculine. In fact, the thought crossed my mind to opt out of this final leg of the journey altogether. My university position was secure, as well as my marriage and finances. I had the cabin to go to when I needed a nature fix and my work to keep me as busy as I wished to stay. I had a wonderful family, and Bud and I had more good friends and entertainment on our plates than we could say grace over.

Yet when the invitation arrived in my mailbox, my heart yearned to dance because it had become clear by then that I had a mission. I was righteously indignant with what dressing up and dancing to the wrong tunes does to women. The tricksters had pushed me too far with their claims that women are incomplete without what they have to offer. And I was sick of heart that I, as well as the vast majority of the women I come in contact with, was suffering with how we look as we age. Thus it was clear that I was being called to action in a way very different from the past. I needed a new way to say the words I wanted to say, go where I needed to go, and meet the people I needed to meet in order to help remedy our plight.

It may seem strange that a professor with a long history of speaking in public and presenting ideas to others would fail to have met her prince earlier. But my high school freshman English teacher didn't address her remarks in my yearbook, "To my quiet, beautiful Karen," for no reason. I, like so many women, shut my authentic voice down early on and let my parlor persona speak for me. And, although I later learned to operate out of my intellect and to talk and write about abstract ideas, I choked when it came to stating how I *felt,* even to close friends. I was especially mute when what I felt in my heart to be true disagreed with what others thought. So the idea of confronting an issue such as positive aging sent me reeling.

I can't say how you will react to the king's invitation. By the time mine arrived, I'd been practicing Native American traditions for some time. So the concept of Great Spirit who is the offspring of Grandmother and Grandfather and whose first two laws are that all is born of woman and that nothing should hurt nature's children was a comfortable place to begin. I again went to the woods where I made a huge pine stump into an altar. Each morning I let the rising sun warm my body, and I burned sage and asked to be granted the privilege of using my voice to speak my midlife truth.

The Festival

The king's festival is an interesting event, for it mirrors both our inner and outer worlds in that the characters and situations we encounter there reflect various aspects of both the psyche and the physical world. For example, those who attended the festival would have worn masks along with their finery. So, when we speak of the festival, we're talking about the false-parlor world and the masked parts of our psyche. But, of course, we know that the two are full of masked players, and that it's now time to go among them undressed of our false-persona and adorned as mature women in the splendid authenticity of our Self.

When Cinderella arrives at the festival, her stepsisters and stepmother don't recognize her. How sad that anyone who isn't masked according to the parlor rules is unrecognizable to them. In their error, they fail to recognize the only maiden in the room who's adorned in authentic beauty.

Likewise, our newly discovered Cinderella is so foreign to our stepsister ego and internal stepmother that they believe our Cinderella beauty has come from a distant land—perhaps another planet. What this means is that as you unmask your authentic appearance, your parlor ego won't be taking hers off simultaneously. So, like the stepmother and sisters, a part of you may feel as though you are in the company of a stranger the first few times you go out sans your old mask.

I recall finding the perfect dress for my stepdaughter's wedding, and, as much as my Cinderella knew that it was authentic, my rational mind told me that it not only didn't look like a mother of the bride dress, it didn't look like anything I'd ever worn before. But I let my Cinderella win out. And sure enough, I didn't look like anyone else at the wedding. But that didn't matter. The dress and I got through the ticklish "blended family" situation with more grace than I would have previously thought possible.

You may also find that your new attitude produces little recognition from family and friends. Stunned looks may cross their faces when you opt out of spiteful conversations about other women's clothing or when they discover that you no longer play one-upmanship with other women's appearance. And why not? Unmasked, you aren't the *you* that they've known all these years, just as Laura wasn't Tim's grammy while she wore her suit.

And changing our personal attitudes about how we look by no means budges other people's old beliefs. They may still have mile-long lists of *shoulds* that are as sacred to them as the commandments on Moses' tablets: Thou shalt not wear sleeveless dresses after thou art forty. Thou shalt not dress different from thy daughter. Thou shalt remove thy wrinkles. Unfortunately, there aren't just ten of *these* commandments. Yet, Cinderella doesn't care that others don't recognize her, and neither do we.

It is important to note that while the stepsisters and stepmother don't recognize Cinderella, they *do* affirm her beauty. What a shift of attitude from when they mockingly called her a little princess after taking away her clothes and abandoning her to the ashy kitchen to now honoring her as a foreign princess! Similarly, even if our own egos and other people don't openly recognize our unmasked, authentic appearance, most of them will respond positively to it on some level. For, when we dress to dance to our own tune with love in our hearts, we meet our conscious self and other people on a higher plane—even those who are still holding tight to their parlor seats.

Dancing with the Prince

Although her family fails to recognize Cinderella, the prince, the one who matters most, certainly perceives her beauty. He's so captivated that he takes her for his partner for the rest of the day. So despite our misgivings, our inner hero responds to our authentic appearance and wants to dance with us.

What does it mean to dance the first day with the prince? It means that we get to know our animus potential. And while this may not sound as romantic as being courted by a real prince, it's every bit as exciting, provocative, mysterious, and magical. Since I've slid on and off the dance floor with more false princes than I care to discuss and didn't want my fear of past failures to mark the most important dance of my life, I asked my therapist to give me a few dance lessons. In a guided visualization, Jeanette carefully brought me to the point where I could meet my inner male animal spirit.

Deep within, I encountered the most magnificent golden tiger in all the world—the ancient symbol of power. But he was so fierce that I pulled back in fright. Jeanette picked up on my vision's energy and sat back too. Since the tiger had now scared both of us, she asked if I wanted to envision putting him in a cage so that he wouldn't be so threatening while I was getting to know him. I didn't want to lock him up, but the strength in that animal was like nothing I had ever experienced.

After a few tentative minutes of his green eyes staring at me and mine staring back at him, I gathered the courage to stroke his side. The tiger was taut. I sensed that he was powerful, and he knew it. What most impressed me was how he held his power. He didn't strut his stuff or fritter it away. In fact, he didn't use it at all. It was enough that we both knew it was there and that he could spring into action at any time.

That was as much as I could take, and Jeanette brought me back into the room. Like Cinderella who wanted to go home when evening came, I couldn't take in the tiger's potency all in one meeting, no matter how handsome and strong he was. He was simply too much. So I turned from him and fled.

We've all experienced this primal urge to fly away from something overwhelmingly powerful in ourselves, be it an animal we meet in a guided meditation or a board meeting where we present a proposal that is adopted unanimously. We accomplish something we set out to do, and at first blush feel good about it. But, then it becomes too overpowering, and we flee.

Before we reconnected to our Selves, as we fled, the internal step-mother would tell us that we were right to run away. She'd convince us that we couldn't repeat the accomplishment, that it wouldn't last, or that it had resulted from luck, which had nothing to do with real ability. She reassured us that we were frauds who would be found out. No wonder we felt like masked impostors.

But now there's a difference in our retreat. We who walk in authentic beauty do as Cinderella does. We understand that ebbing and flowing are innate in women, that backing off and giving ourselves some space is our primal means of integrating our accomplishments. So we leave the festival as evening—the time of the moon—approaches and return to the Mother's tree where we shed our beautiful raiment for the night. Then we take our fears of dancing with the prince and go back to the kitchen. Once again in our gray bedgown, we mull over the day's events and purify them in the ashes. That Cinderella leaves a small lantern on the mantle over the kitchen fireplace is proof positive that her dreams are casting the light of understanding on the events of the day, for light always bespeaks of integration.

It took me more nights among the ashes than I can recount to learn not to fear my inner tiger. Then it took as many more before three messages about his nature became clear. First, the tiger's power was far different from the tyrannical wounded-male, might-makes-right power we're used to, because his potency was neither mean-spirited nor gratuitously violent. Second, the tiger was confident in his own abilities, but his confidence didn't come through vying with others. It was innate.

Finally, the tiger was strangely dispassionate. It was okay that I was there and that I touched his side. He seemed to expect it and probably even liked it. Yet he stayed pretty much into himself. That's because the animus lacks emotion. In his proper role, he is the facilitator and bearer of spirit to our feminine soul, but he cannot *feel*. No wonder we fear meeting our masculine side—we must guard against letting our young, unfeeling, animus rule our egos and run over our fleeing feminine self.

Given this, we retreat to the safety of the inner kitchen for good reason beyond needing to integrate what we've learned so far. It seems that Cinderella's prince isn't yet a knight in shining armor, in that he tries to go home with her to find out to whom she *belongs*. Obviously, he has some lessons to learn about who belongs to whom.

Although he's the son of the good king, the prince has all the makings of a wounded animus. Remember that the masculine principle, like my tiger, lacks emotion. He's all doing, thinking, and reacting. In this dispassionate but highly active state, the animus' drive to accomplish will swamp us in a minute. And if we let him, he'll neither care nor look back. So we must be careful here.

The Developing Animus

Like heroines, young heroes must perform tasks before they are worthy of a royal wedding. And, while it's not my purpose to trace the prince's journey, a few of the tasks that lay ahead of him bear directly on our midlife development.

The first one has to do with the prince's reliance on Cinderella's father, the family's patriarch. After Cinderella escapes, the prince waits until the father passes by and tells him that the strange maiden has slipped into his pigeonhouse. The father muses momentarily about whether the maiden might be Cinderella, but then he asks for an axe and chops the pigeonhouse into a thousand pieces.

That Cinderella's father fails to recognize her comes as no great shock. No one else in her family knows who she is either. But something more than nonrecognition is going on here. We intuit that the father's question is rhetorical, that he knows on some level that the maiden *is* Cinderella.

This is a pivotal point in Cinderella's story as well as our own, for the nonrecognition our authentic beauty receives from our ego and close friends pales in comparison to the outrage created within the larger society by the splendor of the Great Mother that now shines throughout our countenance. The threat to the established order of things that Cinderella imposes when she escapes from the prince and takes refuge in the pigeonhouse, the symbol of the Great Mother's temple, is simply too great for the father to ignore. Inasmuch as destroyed people know only to destroy other people, he razes the birdhouse for the same reason that the old patriarchs pulled down the temples of the goddesses—to rout Her out of his domain.

Had Cinderella invited the prince to go back to the kitchen for a little nookey, things wouldn't have been nearly so dire for the father. He would have faced some social disgrace; however, the prince would have done the honorable thing and married Cinderella because she was so beautiful. Then he would have swamped Cinderella's budding femininity, thereby wounding them both. But Cinderella defies the rules of her father's house. And young maidens who defy the rules are met with sharp instruments of slaughter.

According to Jung, dreams are a direct pipeline to the unconscious, and did mine ever open up after I began my quest to integrate my animus! For six to eight weeks I dreamed of punk teenage boys who tried to wrest my purse at gunpoint. One night I envisioned yellow-furred coyotes (tricksters) trying to catch and eat Maggie, my real-life cocker spaniel who appears in my dreams as my childlike, free spirit. Night after night, dream-men tried to break into my house and stand by my bed and attack me.

We in midlife may find that we dream of losing our teeth or that someone takes our teeth, the symbols of our abilities to bite into things. That we dream of being naked in public testifies to our fear of being seen for who we really are. Some women dream that they are raped or forced to eat food or dirt or feces that they don't want. Others report dreaming that a man or a dark force lives in their basement and will hack them to pieces should they venture too near the cellar door—which, of course, they inevitably do before they wake up in stark terror.

That women who stand at the door of individuation dream these common nightmare themes is far from accidental. Being invaded by the wounded masculine scarred us so deeply that the first layer we encounter when we seek the animus is the chopping the feminine has received over the past six thousand years.

Too, as we move toward developing a positive attitude toward aging and an authentic persona, we may find in our waking hours that others, either men themselves or animus-wounded women, hack at us. A fellow professor opened the door to my office one day after I began writing this book, looked at me in an odd way, and said, "I don't know what you're trying to accomplish! You're an attractive woman. You don't need to make all this fuss."

I was shocked that my work threatened him to the point that he burst into my space and spitefully sliced everything away but my appearance. For sure, it was no compliment. His attack was a swift whack with a double-headed axe. If I weren't attractive, he would have accused me of projecting sour grapes; as it was, he belittled my mission. Although this man's open hostility is rare, the unstated message we get from those like him causes psychic bleeding.

This daily foray into our psyche is mirrored in myriad fairy tales worldwide that involve chopping up fair young maidens. "The Handless Maiden," "Fitcher's Bird," and "Bluebeard" are among hundreds that attest to the reality of our fears of being hacked apart. Yet in each of these, as well as in Cinderella's story, a second attempt is made to reunite the complete feminine with the masculine. So, our fairy tales urge us not to give up, even when our nights are plagued by menacing figures with pickaxes and our days marred by those with scythes for tongues.

Day Two

Armed with the confidence of dancing with the prince on the first day, we again don our sacred symbols and move into the outer world. And just like Cinderella, we glow more brightly because even more light of our inner well-being shines through. And since we no longer need to blindly follow the dictates of others, we have options about how we want to look, and we enjoy the freedom our choices provide.

Generally speaking, if we relish a role because it fits our true calling we enjoy wearing its traditional look. This is normal; there's nothing wrong with wearing an accepted mode if we *want* to, sans the fear and social pressure.

Katy, for example, loves her role as a stay-at-home mother of three high schoolers, and she willingly jumps into T-shirts and jeans when she goes to their various sporting events and puts on silk dresses and heels when she heads to the theater for their opening nights. Several years ago, she bought herself a mother's ring with money she earned from writing articles for a family-oriented magazine. But Katy refuses to wear what she calls "mom clothes"—sweatshirts with "world's greatest mom" or the like on them. To her, these titles commercialize her mission. Too, she doesn't let her children tell her what to wear. She dresses from her personal frame of reference by choosing how *she* wants to look for her primary role of mother.

In addition to eagerly wearing the looks of the roles we particularly enjoy, women often dress for roles that they anticipate taking someday. For example, I see an abrupt change in my women students' appearance at the end of their junior year. As if on cue, they streamline their extreme hair and modify their faddish makeup and clothing in preparation for the job market that they'll enter after graduation.

This tendency to shift our appearance toward the future has major importance to our midlife task. I don't foolishly suggest that we dye our hair gray prematurely, for that's as unnatural as a sixty-five-year-old woman dyeing hers jet black. But we who choose the path of authentic beauty can begin to positively anticipate our inevitable body changes before they occur by observing older women who have aged in mind, body, and soul successfully.

When you see older, beautiful women whom you admire, notice what appeals to you about their appearance. Maybe it's the way they carry themselves or wear their hair. For years I've taken particular note of a shade of gray hair that I think is absolutely beautiful—almost white with a tinge of silver. It shines like a full September moon. Now it looks as if my hair may be turning that very shade. Isn't it amazing how my Mother-given instinct appreciated this shade long before I ever had a silver strand!

The Wrong Fit

While many of our roles and their looks fit like a glove, others don't. If we feel uncomfortably out of place in a role, we'll likely feel strangely unsuited to its mandatory costume. Depending on how much we would like to distance ourselves from a role we don't care for, our feelings about its look will range from mild irritation to outright disgust.

Some resentment against what we *have to* wear is normal, so don't overreact to mild discomforts. Resentment toward our business suit may only mean that we're overworked and need some time away. Not *having* to wear an expected look is what makes weekend and vacation clothes so special. But a persistent, uneasy feeling that we prostitute ourselves when we wear his favorite dress or button up our suit jacket is a red herring— something deeper is amiss.

Perhaps you are an accountant and you deeply value your work, but you aren't too thrilled with having to wear a traditional business suit every day. Maybe you feel that suits restrict your newly found Self. Or suppose you enjoy working for your favorite charity but question the need for wearing expensive evening wear to all those benefit dinners.

Such mildly uncomfortable situations give us a good opportunity to dance with the prince a little. We put our linear thinking cap on, connect it directly to our inner wisdom, and ask them to do a little western two-step entitled "How can I modify my *have to* look so that it reflects more of the real me?" Once you open your heart and ask this question, then answers float around you like Cinderella's dresses. You come to understand that even though you must look a way that doesn't express enough of the real you, you can wear *something* expressive.

A friend who's in a very powerful business position wears subtle spirit-animal jewelry—gold wolves and sterling silver eagles—right into the boardroom, and no one is the wiser to their spiritual nature. Why not wear a scandalously risqué teddy or cotton boxer shorts with big red lips under your lab coat? What a way to tickle your fancy. When you make such seemingly insignificant changes that reflect *you,* the benefits are monumental, because you come away liking your roles so much more and are better at performing them. So, in treating your Cinderella self to what it likes, those around you benefit from your productivity and temperament, too.

Another way to handle less-than-comfortable looks is to barter with yourself. Tell yourself, I have no choice but to buy evening clothes if I want to support this worthwhile charity. But from now on I'll buy less, wear it more often, and for each dress I buy, I'll buy a new pair of jeans and a sweater (or whatever fits your style).

Ah-ha, now you've struck a deal with your various roles, one that really works. Because when you barter, each of your multifaceted parts feels unafraid that you'll sell it out for another. And as you'll soon see, keeping your multifaceted Self balanced is paramount to your ability to dance.

Also try reevaluating your *have to* situations. Are there times when you can negotiate with a look in some way? Can you wear jeans to work when no clients will be there to see you? Must you wear a strictly pared-down business look, or can you modify it somewhat? Prod around to discover if there's some slack (*bad* pun). Sometimes we go on automatic pilot and don't really explore all our possibilities. Check yours out. I'll bet there's more room to express your Self than you think.

Remember that feeling uncomfortable about a look doesn't give you specific direction as to *where* your discomfort lies. Too often we project negative feelings onto our appearance, because, if we faced our ambivalence toward the role itself, we'd be forced to admit that we're uncomfortable with it.

For example, if you truly hate your business suits but claim to love being an attorney, you need to do some serious soul searching. I wouldn't be convinced for a minute that your dislike for your suits is merely a reaction to their styling or colors. My gut feeling would be that you're unhappy with your role and are superficially clinging to the belief that your professional choice is the right one but that something dire is wrong with its appropriate look.

Perhaps as you mull over the situation when you return to the kitchen at night, you'll recognize that the only reason you became a lawyer is because your father was a lawyer—that you acted out the good little girl role for him and cast aside your true desire to become a commercial artist. While this revelation may be hard to accept, it will put you on the track to correcting a serious rift within yourself.

Severe incongruities between our roles and the way we look while playing them are much more than mere irritations. Our true Self cannot operate when our appearance and roles are at each other's throats; the split leaves too bloody a gash. Corrective action is in order here, whether it be as serious as a full career change or merely that you enroll in a drawing class at the local YWCA.

I can't overstress that when it comes to the appropriateness of our roles, our appearance "voice" is steady and true. Since it comes from that place of deepest knowing in our Self, it won't lie to us. So, when you return to sleep by the kitchen fire each evening, ask the good Mother for guidance as you assess your roles. Be open to what your white bird tells you. Look closely at those areas where feelings about what you do and how you dress while doing it differ radically. These differences are clues that you may not be reaching your full potential, that you are acting out a role that violates your Self, or that you're still trying to dance to other people's tunes.

More Chopping

As he had the evening before, the prince waits for the father to pass by and informs him that the maiden eluded him and climbed into the pear tree. This time the father symbolically casts the Great Mother asunder by chopping away Her life's force. Axing down a pear tree, whose womb-shaped fruit has stood for the mystical feminine since the beginning of time, bespeaks of the length and breath the patriarchy goes to maintain supremacy.

We certainly see a backlash against the current rise of the feminine spirit as our leaders chop away equal opportunity legislation and in the

202 — Positive Aging

increased woman bashing by such notables as Howard Stern and Rush Limbaugh. But perhaps the most poignant recent testimony to society's disdain of the complete feminine was the volcano of emotions that spewed forth as a result of the murders of Nicole Brown Simpson and Ronald Goldman and the subsequent trial of O. J. Simpson.

If we scratch beneath the sordid surface, we find that the characters mirror the archetypes of the hero who pines for his true love, the fair-haired maiden who seeks to go out on her own, the golden boy who tries to help her, and the murderer who ends her budding independence by chopping her up. That the accused meter of death and justice was a quintessential national sports hero, complete with all the wounded masculine characteristics society so admires in its heroes—money, fame, physical prowess, good looks, and magnetic personality—the story becomes spooky in its symbolism. Then when the trickster, Mark Fuhrman, surfaced late in the case and bungled the evidence against the hero so badly that he was set free, our morning newspapers took on the aura of a Homeric epic.

My point has nothing to do with whether or not Mr. Simpson did or didn't kill his ex-wife. The issue is the extent to which society perceived the characters archetypally and concentrated on the tragic hero figure, while for the most part overlooking the fact that a beautiful young woman and her friend were murdered.

But we must not let the father have his way. Cinderella escapes a second time by shimmying up a pear tree like a squirrel, the collector of nuts. Nuts, as we know, stand for the wisdom of the crone and the potential within the maiden. So Cinderella is again strengthened by ancient wisdom as she as escapes back to the ashy sanctuary of the kitchen for another night of dreams. For even though her father attacked the pear tree, she cannot let him keep her from dancing with the prince on the following day.

Day Three

By the last day of the festival, getting to know our animus has become so important to our journey that we're all but oblivious to society's messages about youth and fashion. Like the prince who keeps Cinderella away from all other dance partners, our maturing masculine energy protects us from being lured away from him. Yes, we hear the commercials for antiaging products and good-naturedly listen to our friends recount the merits of having chin-lifts, but ads and others' *shoulds* hold little chance of luring us off course because we know with whom we're dancing and why.

On this final day, we fox-trot to the tune that opens us up to the realization that we are multidimensional women and that each part of us embodies a power that we'll need in our upcoming season. As we step to the tempo, we explore how to give expression to each part through our appearance.

Unfortunately, the father's parlor has provided little room for exploring our multiselves. Instead, as little girls we were taught to cling to a single definition of who we are. So, for most of our lives, we've lived out but one of our many sides, regardless of the number of roles we play.

If we've viewed ourselves primarily as a sexual persona, for example, our entire wardrobe reflects it, like Andrea and Barbara in Chapter Seven. Barbara's look is that of a sexy little girl whether she's working at her office or attending a barbecue—just what we'd expect her to look like as she plays the singular role of her husband's sex kitten. Andrea, on the other hand, plays the eternal femme fatale. Whether she's teaching a class or taking a bunch of kids to the park, she wears the same call girl look.

Other women play the socialite exclusively, regardless of what they are doing or with whom. They costume themselves solely from an actor's trunk filled with name-brand designers and pricey jewelry.

However, a sexy-looking or bejeweled professional woman cuts her chances of playing out her role credibly and thereby hamstrings her chances for raises and promotions. On the other hand, who wants to go to bed with someone who never dons anything other than something from the pages of a Brooks Brothers catalog, or attend a gala event with a woman who tries to make an appearance-related political statement regardless of the occasion? When we assume such singular identities, we smother all but one of our valuable and beautiful selves, because refusing to acknowledge that we're anything but a mother, a sexy woman, a woman with a political stance, or a daughter of a well-known family is stifling.

To do ourselves and our roles justice, we need to develop what I call a "Meryl Streep" approach to what we wear. Chief among the qualities that makes Ms. Streep one of the greatest actresses of our time is her ability to immerse herself fully in each role and bring to life each character's idiosyncrasies and unique personality. Remember how differently she portrayed the women in *Sophie's Choice* and *The Bridges of Madison County?* When you think of it, our roles are as diverse as hers, because being a sexy wife requires a very different attitude and wardrobe than being a teacher.

That each of our multiple selves desires to blossom and be adorned uniquely, however, doesn't mean that we will end up fracturing our personalities. Quite the opposite, our goal is to integrate the various parts of our psyches and at the same time give voice to our multifaceted talents, interests, and activities. Rather than being at odds with ourselves, we really can unveil all the fascinating women who dwell within us without playing the lead role in *The Three Faces of Eve*.

Jung's protégé, Toni Wolff, developed the framework for integrating and expressing our various parts back in the 1930s when she outlined four basic types of female personality patterns based on four Greek goddess types. However, before we look at them, let me first say that I'm suspect of linking women's personalities primarily to one goddess or another. Although we surely gain insight by studying the mythological heroines and incorporating their characteristics into our daily lives, we need to be cir-

cumspect that in so doing we don't get boxed into even greater uni-
dimensionality.

Too, an even bigger stumbling block exists in some of the goddess literature in that several well-known authorities (whom I otherwise greatly
respect) fail to recognize the full nature of beauty when they relate it only
to Aphrodite. Unfortunately, this limits beauty to a single realm and rein-
forces aging stereotypes. Let's not forget that Paris so enraged Hera and
Athena when he awarded the golden apple to Aphrodite for being the
most beautiful that he caused the never-to-be-forgotten Trojan War. It
seems that each goddess thought that *she* was the fairest in the land—and
so do the various female archetypes in us.

With that caveat, let's look at Wolff's model. She labeled the four
major types of female subpersonalities: Mother, Amazon, Hetaira, and
Medium. She presented them as being part of a circle, because they are
connected to one another. The Mother is at the top of the circle and the
Hetaira is at the bottom. The Medium is to the left, and the Amazon is on
the right.

The Mother, which we might associate with the goddess Demeter,
places her highest value on her family. She's like my neighbor Katy whose
greatest joy comes from raising her children. At her best, she brings love
and nurturance to the world. At her worst, she is the devourer.

The Amazon places greatest priority on her self-sufficiency and independence. These women are fathers' daughters, inasmuch as they, like
Athena, patterned themselves on the active masculine rather than on the
traditional feminine. They often serve as role models regarding how to
make it in the physical world, but without some balance they can become
unfeeling tyrants.

Hetaira's nature is sensual and may exude sexuality, as did Aphrodite,
in that female sexuality is one with our potent creative force. These
women abound in the arts. However, the undeveloped Hetaira limits herself to playing out either the role of sexy woman or muse for men. And,

when she falls short of her potential to create for herself, she becomes a self-destructive demon.

The Medium corresponds to Persephone and Hecate and resides in the spirit realm of the unconscious. In Native American tradition, this would be the West where ancient feminine wisdom and the Great Mystery lie. Women who traverse their inner self easily and instinctively and trust their intuition are in tune with the Medium. However, carried to the extreme, they become moody, dreamy, and ineffective in the physical world.

A major part of the process of individuation is incorporating and balancing all four archetypes within our psyches, to bring them to consciousness so that they can help us carry out our roles. For, if we fail to breathe life into them, they will lie in the shadow of our unconscious and create the havoc that unrecognized parts have a way of doing.

Integrating the four isn't easy, however. On introspection, we may find that we're partial to one type—we have no trouble seeing how the Amazon or Hetaira influences our life, for example. And it's not so difficult to recognize and integrate the two types that lie adjacent to our primary type because in one way or another they share some common traits. But we often have *major* problems dealing with the type that lies directly across the circle from our primary one.

For example, as a classic Hetaira, I'm ever-so-much more at home in her role as well as those that call forth my Medium and Amazon aspects. However, I struggled for years to learn how to accommodate the Mother in me. In my failure to integrate her, I inadvertently played out the role of evil stepmother to my stepchildren, friends, family, students, and coworkers. From out of nowhere, it seemed, I'd be overtaken by an invisible force and turned into a shrew. Thus, I wasn't too surprised that during my first attempt at active imagination Snow White's stepmother appeared front and center in my mind. She'd been anonymously calling the shots from my shadow for more than forty years and had more to say about being shoved back than I have space here to recount. Yet even today, after trying my best to integrate the full range of Mother, operating out of the other three types is still much more to my primary nature.

Although it may be somewhat uncomfortable, however, incorporating these four feminine types empowers us to play our roles with greater ease and effectiveness. Without integrating them, we either live compartmentalized or fragmented lives. Barbara and Andrea, as I've said, compartmentalized themselves into a sexy-woman role somewhere along the way. Others try to knit together seemingly separate roles, such as mother and actress, and often find themselves asking again and again "Who am I?"

The ambiguity we feel from having multiple roles is called role conflict. It can come from others, such as when Tim refuses to acknowledge Laura's professional life. Or it may be a personal ambivalence over how to fit our many roles into our hectic lives. Regardless of the cause, however, role conflict is serious business. The discomfort can sap our abilities to play any of our roles out to their fullest.

Laura, the attorney we met in the last chapter, has a daughter, Debra, who is a single mom living in Atlanta. She and Laura have worked out an agreement whereby Tim visits Laura in Seattle for a month each year. Having a whole month together gives Tim and Laura a chance to get to know each other and Debra some personal space. But because of her practice, Laura can't take the month off when Tim visits, so she hires a teenager to stay with him.

When Laura puts on her suit each morning during Tim's visit, she feels both pride and an uneasy twinge, because she's torn between two competing needs. She's pulled between maintaining her high professional performance (Athena) and feeling guilty over leaving Tim with a caretaker (Mother). Her sweats bespeak of the good times she and Tim have after work and on weekends. But they also attest to her inability to see Rick, her lover, as often and under the circumstances she would like (Hetaira). Similarly, the clothes Laura wears with Rick are so different from those she wears while working in her garden that he teases her about them. Yet her garden is important, because it's the place she goes to commune with nature and be with her Self (Medium).

We can see each of the feminine forms at work here; and, unless she gets a handle on it, Laura's role conflict is akin to Paris' beauty contest—a push and pull for supremacy that results in all-out war. And truly, that's what role conflict can amount to if we aren't centered. We're pulled from stem to stern by every person and circumstance that has a claim on us. And our animus, like the heroes and gods whom the warring goddesses finally turned against each other and ultimately weakened, is rendered ineffective.

Once Laura reconnected to her Self and learned to dress from her heart, however, she began to get the upper hand over her internal and external conflicts. She recognized the fact that she cannot dress for her competing needs and the persons in her life all at the same time—she's simply incapable of dancing to four tunes at once. Too, she understood that others' demands on her cannot and should not rule how she divides her energies. Despite Rick's misgivings about her need to spend time in her garden alone and Tim's inability to understand why she goes to her office instead of staying with him, these are necessary parts of her that must be honored.

What she discovered is that dressing for each of her roles pays off tenfold. Her various outfits help her to focus full attention on what she needs to *at the moment*. So, when she honors her Athena side and puts on her suit, she puts on her attorney attitude and abilities along with it. When she mulches her flower beds while wearing old sweaters and jeans, she gives no thought to what she and Rick will have for dinner that evening. She remains balanced, because she's careful to give each part of herself a good measure of undivided time and attention. While this doesn't keep either Tim or Rick from demanding more than she can give to them at times, it removes 90 percent of the guilt and confusion from her multifaceted life.

Facing the Truth

In *The Woman's Dictionary of Symbols and Sacred Objects,* Barbara Walker refers to the adage that, "The Devil is the curse of those who have abandoned the Goddess." If we view Cinderella's father's destructive actions in light of this, we intuit that he eventually will be made a fool of. And indeed, the father makes a buffoon of himself, for both times he tries to help the prince, Cinderella eludes him long before he comes on the scene.

So by the third day, the prince has learned a very valuable lesson—the one that ultimately renders him fit for the daughter of the good mother. The old father is of no value to him, and he must catch the illusory maiden himself.

The prince's lesson is valuable for us, too. For, at this point, we are strong and wise enough to face a major truth—that the patriarchy is of no value to us in our quest for positive aging and authentic appearance. Shortly before I began collecting my thoughts for this chapter, I had the following dream that put the whole issue into perspective:

I'm in a houseboat with a man, and we prepare to fish. I throw my line out a window into the ocean and immediately feel a ferocious tug. I'm elated at the thought of catching a big fish. But my joy turns to stark terror as I look out and see three fins rising up out of the water and then a ten- to twelve-foot shark turning and racing straight toward me.

The shark rages furiously because I snared him in the back and brought him to the surface. I stop reeling him in. But he keeps on rushing toward me to eat me—his huge mouth open, exposing hundreds of flashing teeth.

I have to let him go, and I turn to ask the man to cut the line for me. But he's no longer there, and I must sever it myself. I try to break the fishing line with my fists, thinking all the while that you can't pull fish wire apart. Yet I am so scared of the wild, thrashing shark that I keep pulling until I break the line, and the shark disappears back into the ocean.

In probably no more than a minute or two, the dream presented a panoramic picture of the last 6000 years. Rather than catch a fish, the ancient symbol of the sensual goddess, I had reached into my unconscious and snared the male trinity (the three fins) giving steerage to sharklike aggressiveness. Not only had I brought the shark up to the surface, but in doing so I had exposed it for the beast that it is. The wounded masculine was furious and was coming to gobble me up for dislodging it from its comfortable realm in the unconscious where it rules as the undisputed king and forages on whatever and whomever it chooses. This monster from the deep, in itself, was frightening enough. But I soon discovered to my horror that I could not get help from the man, the symbol of our society. *I must sever my line to the three-finned shark myself.*

So with all the strength we can muster in our bare hands—our symbolic means of grasping life and acting out our creativity—we must sever the line that has linked us with the wounded-masculine tenets, behaviors, and emotions that have held us to the old ways of conceiving female beauty and aging. As we do, we know full well that we can't do much personally to rout the beast from society-at-large. But at least when we've made peace in our own hearts with our appearance, we're enabled to dress and carry ourselves in a manner that allows us to live authentic lives.

The True Prince

Once he separates himself from Cinderella's father, the prince is independent to act on his own. Once independent, he's worthy to be the king's son and ready to unite with the daughter of the true mother. He proves that when he uses pitch, a fossil fuel that symbolizes his natural energy, to snare Cinderella's slipper. In other versions, the prince uses honey to hold the slipper—an ancient symbol of the powerfully feminine queen bee.

It's also significant that Cinderella's left slipper got stuck; the left symbolizing the inner, intuitive, receptive side of our psyches. Thus, we

know that the prince has integrated a certain amount of the loving feminine, a rounding-out he needed as much as Cinderella needed to incorporate some of the activating masculine before either are fit for the royal
marriage.

The good mother herself knew that the prince was ready for
Cinderella, too. Instead of slippers the color of the moon and embroidered with silk, on the third day they shone of the king's gold.

The glass slippers worn by Cinderella in alternative versions of the
story also speak to us who travel the midlife journey. Glass connotes the
clarity we seek by integrating the masculine and the feminine, but at the
same time our inability to reach out and take it—for Cinderella and the
prince aren't wed yet. Glass frequently symbolizes this transparent barrier
in other fairy tales of integration such as "Snow White," wherein the prince
finds Snow White in a glass coffin, and "The Seven Ravens," where the
maiden locates her bewitched brothers inside a glass mountain. In each,
the object of the character's desire lays behind glass, out of immediate
grasp.

The prince cannot reach out and grasp us, because, although he may
be sure of us, we're still not so sure about him. Again we escape and run
back down the stairway, *down* into the realm of our good Mother. Yes, we
can dance pretty well now, and we trust the prince. We're even fond of
him. But we remain a stranger in the territory of the festival, because even
as we wear our radiant dresses and golden shoes we continue to feel vulnerable. In this in-between stage, it's best that we again return home to
Mother, give back our dress and our remaining gold slipper, and spend one
more night nestled by the warm kitchen fire.

But the prince won't give up. As Cinderella hurries back to the hazel
tree and then on to the sanctuary of the kitchen, he picks up her tiny
golden slipper and vows to find the mysterious maiden to whom it
belongs. Thus, with the plot set and the cast in place, the stage is set for
the final act.

Meeting Your Inner Women

To help integrate the various feminine archetypes in yourself, go within
and find out how each—Mother, Hetaira, Athena, and Medium—feels
about your attitudes, activities, and appearance. And don't slight one
because she seems foreign or abhorrent. Take her to tea some afternoon
and ask her what she enjoys doing and how she wants to look doing it.
Does she have a favorite color? She may prove to be that inner voice that
comes out of nowhere who repeatedly asks for a Victoria's Secret catalog
or a backpack. Listen to her, and then wear whatever she suggests when
you slip into her role.

　　Rest assured, now that you're no longer at the mercy of whatever
comes flying up at you from your unconscious, a splintered-off type can't
remake either your life or your appearance when you bring her into consciousness; she'll only swamp you with guilt and ineffectiveness if you
ignore her. Balance and empower your Self by letting the four feminine
forms express themselves through your appearance.

The ultimate marriage of spirit and soul, ani-
mus and anima, *is the wedding of heaven and*
earth, our highest ideals and ambitions united
with our lowliest symptoms and complaints.

—Thomas Moore, *Care of the Soul*

Ten

The Royal Wedding:
Positive Aging

The next morning the prince took the shoe to the father and said, "I shall wed she
whose foot fits this golden slipper." This pleased the two stepsisters, for they had
pretty feet.

The eldest took the shoe into her room to try it on, but she couldn't get her big
toe into it. Then her mother gave her a knife and said, "Cut the toe off; as Queen thou
wilt have no more need to walk." The maiden cut the toe off, forced her foot into the
shoe, and swallowed the pain. The prince took her on his horse as his bride, and they
rode off. However, as they passed the mother's grave, two pigeons who sat in the
hazel tree cried,

"Turn and peep, turn and peep,
There's blood in the shoe,
The shoe it is too small,
The true bride waits for you."

The prince saw the blood and turned his horse around and took the false bride back to her home. The other sister went into her chamber to try on the shoe, but her heel was too big. So her mother gave her the knife and said, "Cut a bit off thy heel; as Queen thou wilt have no need to go on foot." So the maiden sliced a piece off her heel, forced it into the shoe, and swallowed the pain. But as the prince and second stepsister passed the tree, the pigeons again cried that there was blood in the shoe.

The prince saw blood running out of her shoe, staining her white stocking. Then he turned the horse around and took the second false bride home.

"Have you no other daughter?" the prince asked. "No," said the man, "There is a little stunned kitchen wench that my late wife left behind, but she cannot be the bride." The king's son asked to have her sent, but the mother answered, "Oh no, she is much too dirty!" Yet when the prince insisted, Cinderella was summoned.

Cinderella first washed her face and hands and then went to the king's son and took the golden shoe. She seated herself on a stool, drew her foot from the wooden clog, and put it into the slipper. When she stood, the prince looked at her face and recognized the beautiful maiden who had danced with him and cried, "She is the true bride!"

The stepmother and sisters were terrified and paled with rage; he, however, took Cinderella on his horse. As they passed the tree, the two white doves cried,

"Turn and peep, turn and peep,

No blood is in the shoe,

The shoe's just right,

The true bride rides with you."

They swooped down and sat on Cinderella's shoulders, one on the right, the other on the left.

As time approached for the royal wedding, the two false sisters wanted to gain Cinderella's favor so they could share in her good fortune. On the way to the church, the elder was at the couple's right side and the younger at the left, and the pigeons pecked out one eye from each of them. Afterward as they came back, the elder was at the left, and the younger at the right, and the pigeons pecked out the other eye from each. And thus, for their evil and falsehood, they were punished with blindness.

It would seem that Cinderella and the prince have been through enough, that the final interference from the stepmother and old father is undue. But we, like they, must overcome, not merely sidestep, two of society's most pervasive and powerful archetypes. And, since they are rooted deeply in our unconscious and may still have a grip on our ego, they aren't routed easily. Thus, the final events are crucial if we are to undress our former reliance on youthful beauty and elitist fashion and empower ourselves with authentic appearance.

From the point in the story where the prince comes for his bride, all the way through the royal wedding, we see the classic format of a rite of passage, the ceremony of death to the old and rebirth into the new that allows us to move forward. Given that we have no structure for midlife rites such as were part of every woman's experience in days of old, the model presented in this last part of Cinderella's story is crucial.

Although I use the story of Cinderella as the framework for the rite of passage that will send you on your way to age positively and walk in authentic beauty, I'm not proposing a *specific* ceremony. The particulars of your rite will avail themselves as you work to separate from the wounded father and the Dark Mother and ride off with your inner prince.

In times gone by, women would have gone into the mountains and deserts in groups for rites of passage. Even though they lived close to the earth, it was requisite that they leave the village and go to sacred places for such a time. If we wish to claim the essential feminine, we may want to do likewise, thereby re-creating the ancient community of women who supported each other as they aged. So, as part of your ceremony, you may want to attend one of the many workshops that offer general rites of passage into midlife at rustic sites. If a ceremony to honor midlife beauty isn't part of the ritual, incorporate your own. Most group leaders welcome such personal input. Who knows? Your suggestion to include authentic beauty might prove meaningful to other women as well.

Perhaps you'll choose to create your own rite and perform it with close friends in a nearby woods or in someone's backyard. As part of your ceremony, you might include a birth reenactment or baptism in water or smoke. The possibilities are endless because there are no rules save one. Given that rites of passage are communal in nature, that they involve caring and concerned others, I suggest that you not conduct a ceremony by yourself unless you honestly feel that you cannot share your newly developed understanding of midlife spirit and beauty with others. And under no circumstances would you want to go into nature alone and conduct a rite that would endanger you in any way.

Regardless of your particular ceremony, however, call on your inner wisewomen, child, and spirit animals or inner essences to assist you. Ask the Goddess to join you—especially Her crone manifestations such as Hecate, Spider Grandmother, or Sarah. Invite your female ancestors to be with you.

Dying to the Past

In the first stage of a rite of passage a woman is separated from her old life. Symbolically, she dies to it. At this point in the story, Cinderella is certainly dead and buried to her former existence because the events of the past three days severed her from all that she had known before. Neither her stepfamily nor her father recognize her for who she really is, thus she's as invisible to them as if she'd never existed. Too, for the three days she left the refuge of her mother's grave and went to the palace of the king. As she danced with the prince, she experienced life in a manner unknown to the kitchen's all-feminine inner world. Now she's a different person from the young maiden who first asked for gold and silver to be thrown down to her. How she must question the turn of events as she goes about her morning chores.

So it is with us as we journey forward into the final leg of adorning our Self. When we severed ourselves from the parlor, we discovered so much about our appearance and the mighty role it can play in our autumn.

Then, readorned in our Mother's beauty, we moved into the light of day and danced with our newly discovered life's force. But now the time has come to sit and wait for the unknown that lies ahead—for we still don't quite know how everything is going to work out.

That's because Cinderella isn't the only one who plays a role in our ritual. The family also bears heavily in this final scenario. As the events of the morning unfold, the family acts out the sequence of emotions that precedes impending death: denial, anger, bargaining, depression, and acceptance. And for certain, parts our psyche, like the family, now sense a death to the old ways and react accordingly.

True and False

True to their nature, Cinderella's family remains firm in their unwillingness to acknowledge Cinderella's true identity by denying her existence. Instead, the oldest stepsister who had asked for beautiful dresses when the father went to the fair asks for the slipper. It's paradoxical but prophetic that this parlor sitter takes the shoe to the privacy of her bedroom, for she knows full well she's not the true bride.

The part of our stepsister ego who has banked on our youthful appearance all these years also knows at this juncture that she's an impostor. But, rather than be dethroned, she tries with all her might to fit into the golden slipper. As in Cinderella's story, after the festival, our activating animus may be tempted by our stepsister ego. For just when we think that our authentic Self can now shine forth into the world in its true raiment, the parlor-sitting ego attempts with all her might to convince us that her false appearance is worthy of the true prince—that we should *deny* this stupid notion that her type of beauty is injurious to our upcoming season.

My stepsister desire for youthful beauty tried to take control as my fiftieth birthday loomed ever closer. Even though I'd worked for several years to confront my ego's addiction to my earlier looks and discover my authentic appearance, as July melted into August, the thought of October shrouded me in dread of my autumn season, and I resisted having to acknowledge the end of my summer—once and for all. Repeatedly I asked myself, "Didn't my youthful looks get me thus far? . . . Good grief, look at all I was able to do with them—more than most and then some . . . What if I don't want to use the power of my second half? . . . Maybe I can still accomplish what I'm supposed to without all this hullabaloo." But there was no denying the pull of the upcoming season, and the truth was that the little golden shoe simply didn't fit my big fat ego.

At the thought of her eldest daughter not wedding the prince, the stepmother becomes angry, the second stage in the grieving process. Then she lets loose the full force of her vile and deadly nature. And we, too, are capable of throwing quite a tantrum.

When I finally realized that trying to overlook my need to let go of my former looks was getting me nowhere, I became furious. "Are you nuts? What are you really getting from this positive aging stuff? . . . *Nothing!* And you're trying to teach other women about it . . . *What a hoot!*" But after listening to my hysterical Dark Mother rant for as long as I could take it, I finally calmed down, whereupon I entered the third stage of the grieving process. I began to bargain.

Handing her daughter a knife, the stepmother told her to cut the toe off, saying that when she became queen she wouldn't need it. Like Cinderella's stepsister, I listened to the Dark Mother tell me that if the golden slipper doesn't fit, all I have to do is *modify* my previous dependency on youthful attractiveness and everything will go on splendidly for me. She began to whisper, "Go ahead and have those cosmetic surgeries and take off the *extra* pounds." She tried to soothe my fears by telling me that I wouldn't be hampered in my midlife growth once I'd consummated the royal union. "Just think how good you'll look while you accomplish the mission of your second half," she cackled. "And that old toe? You won't even miss it!"

Tell-Tale Blood

We get a powerful message when the prince and the eldest stepsister pass the hazel tree and two pigeons cry of the false bride and her bloody shoe. It takes me back to my grandmother's knee—the mighty matriarchal knee of my father's family—where I was first introduced to the Brothers Grimm and their tales of heroines, heroes, and evil deeds. Now a retired speech teacher, she performed this passage as though it were the role of a lifetime. And I shivered in its imagery, as she rolled out, "There's *blllooood* on the shoe!"

I shiver to this day for good reason, far beyond the drama that was conjured up in a five year old by a talented grandmother. Despite what our inner stepmother tells us, we cannot hack off our big toe without dire consequences. For when we slice flesh away, life's blood is sacrificed.

It's significant that two birds now sit in the mother's tree and that they call down to the prince. He has danced with Cinderella and shaken off the potential of being contaminated by the wounded father, so he's as intuitively attuned to the birds as is Cinderella. Pigeons are messengers of the divine to the masculine as well as the feminine, because they symbolize home and family. And true to their mission, they cry out a warning to the prince so he won't carry a false bride back to his castle.

As our parlor-ego bargains to retain her supremacy even as we attempt to unite with the spirit-bearing masculine, our birds will alert us before we act if we but listen to them and then heed their advice. In *Parabola*'s 1980 issue on women, editor Lorraine Kisly urges the woman who chooses to remake herself to ask, "How what she chooses to do relates to her being a woman. What will isolate and alienate her from her own nature and from others? What will help connect her to herself and support her search on all levels?"

If we ask our intuitive birds these questions as the stepmother urges us to cut off our big toe, we'll know in a split-second that she's as wrong as she can be about not needing our toe when we become queen. The birds help us realize that regardless of the stakes, a bargain with the devil is no bargain at all.

In every story since the beginning of time, when humans bargain with the evil one, they give up far more than they gain. And, in fairy tales where a false bride is first fostered onto the king's son, the false bride's desire to unite with him is so great that she's willing to destroy any and all who get in her way, for she knows only of destruction and nothing of genuine love.

And what are the stakes here? The eldest stepdaughter has to swallow the pain her mother inflicts on her, for the amputation isn't without side effects. The outcome of slicing off a big toe is the loss of balance. In other words, the part of our complex-plagued ego who still wants to rely on youthful beauty is perfectly willing to render us unbalanced, out of sync with the Self, in order to maintain status quo.

Yet, we need the balance of an uncompromised Self to raise the queen, the mature Cinderella, to the forefront of our consciousness as we age into our mid-years. The queen is the highest form of the complete feminine. She is the Goddess, herself, who must remain vital and in equilibrium in order to inspire our creativity and hold a place for spirit to touch it with the divine spark.

More Blood

The younger stepsister wasn't able to get her heel into the slipper, so the stepmother handed her the knife. Whereas the eldest daughter tried to bargain with youthful beauty, a commodity we know isn't really ours to keep, the second daughter, the one who holds dear the clout of a wounded power-based appearance, might appear to be an even better match for our mighty internal hero. And, indeed, some women turn themselves into privileged, power-mongering queens as they age.

But what might seem at first blush to be a match made in heaven casts us into a living hell, because the heel we're forced to cut off is the most vulnerable part of our foot. If we cut off our heel, we're as subject to a deadly attack as was Achilles, whose mother was unable to coat his heel when she dipped him into a protective potion. When Paris' arrow pierced it, Achilles died. As heels are our primary means of connecting with the Great Mother's earth, anything that hinders us from coming into contact with Her soon bleeds us dry of nourishment and protection.

Too, we know from the father's example what happens to those who try to fool the Goddess. Sooner or later they're made a fool of. If we fall victim to the Dark Mother's assertion that as well-clad queens we won't need to walk, we'll only get as far as the Mother's tree before the birds once again sing of bloody slippers and false brides. Not only will the tiny slipper be filled with the blood of our wounded ego, but our stocking will run red with the sacrifice we made in the name of social and economic elitism.

Philosopher and Eastern culture specialist R. H. Blyth is quoted in *Parabola* as saying that we should strive for "agedness" rather than "oldness" in that oldness is "dryness and decline of life and energy," where as "agedness" lacks stupidity, insensitiveness, egotism, and cruelty, that agedness is without "cynicism, obstinacy, and pride of power." This is a potent description of the difference between the outcomes of the marriage between the prince and the second false bride and the authentic royal union that will carry us through our second half.

The True Bride

Given a little space in our soul and trust in our heart, our prince will find us, just as the prince found the true bride. His intuition is intact and functioning—he *knows* that another maiden lives in the father's house. And by now he's stronger than the old father and stepmother even though they cry in protest against him meeting the child of the good mother. So he demands that Cinderella be summoned.

When called, Cinderella washes her face and hands and ascends the stairs to the parlor. In this, she enters the *albedo*, the white stage in the alchemical process. wherein transformation takes place. As such, she emerges from the kitchen as a new being who will soon enter into a wholly different life from that which she has known previously.

We who sit ready to be reborn into a new consciousness of positive aging are dirty and bloody from our stay in the *negredo* and *rubedo* of the grave-womb. Our unwashed condition bespeaks of tuning out the world and its cosmetic pretenses and working in the ashy kitchen, and it symbolizes our days at the Mother's tree. Before we ascend into the daylight of our new life, we, like Cinderella, seek cleansing baptismal waters. For example, those who participate in formal rites of passage often find that although they may have fasted for many hours prior to the final ritual, when they are brought into the group for the final time, their instincts aren't to eat but to wash their faces and comb their hair—to clean themselves so that they can walk back into the light of the circle. The cleansing ritual is so important, in fact, that many rites incorporate it into the ceremony itself.

Although I didn't participate in a formal rite of passage as I approached my dreaded fiftieth birthday, I found that standing in the shower and letting the water run over me was strangely soothing. My close friend Fran built an outdoor shower and spent night after night washing away her fears about aging under Mother's moon. Her experience was so life affirming that I followed suit and built one in my yard, too.

Despite our ego's misgivings, however, at this crucial point in our journey toward positive aging that virginal part of us that knows the truth about authentic appearance is now ready to leave the kitchen and walk into the light of day, because she has no more reason to be sequestered. It may not dawn on us all at once, but as another friend Gretchen said sometime after her fiftieth birthday, "After all the months of anguish, it finally came to me that I just am who I am, and people are going to have to accept me like this."

And what of our appearance? Cinderella comes up from the kitchen of the unconscious into the light of the parlor and sits down to try on the slipper in full view of all who are present because she knows it will fit. And, as our authentic appearance comes into full view of all, we have no need to explain our Selves to anyone, either. We have undressed the old guilt and shame that came from believing that how we look was subject to other's scrutiny. I'm reminded of a story Oprah Winfrey related to *Ebony*: "The other day I was jogging down the road and this woman said to me, 'You better quit losing so much weight because you're going to make the rest of us feel bad.' What she really meant was, 'Listen, if you start looking better than I do, I'm not going to like you anymore.' Well, I'm finally ready to own my own power, to say, 'All right, this is who I am. If you like it, you like it. And if you don't, you don't. So watch out. I'm gonna fly.'"

In preparation to fly away with the prince, Cinderella takes off her heavy wooden clog, then she places her little foot once again into the golden slipper. Historically, rites of passage have incorporated ritually removing clothing that is symbolic of the old stage and readorning the body in that which bespeaks of the new. Recently, I received a brochure for a women's spirituality workshop that required each participant to bring an article of clothing to be ritually sacrificed and another to don as a symbol of new awareness of spirit. In some ceremonies, removal of the old clothing precedes the cleansing ceremony. Then the new, spirit-filled garment is draped about the novitiate's body so that she walks into her new life symbolically clad for her new role.

When we allow the virgin to ascend the stairs, clean up her little smudged face, remove her heavy wooden shoes, and readorn her in her rightful splendor, our animus recognizes her for the true bride that she is. We can feel this powerful recognition in ourselves when it takes place. When we put on the right garment or piece of jewelry for the right mood or occasion, we feel a powerful "click," and we know for sure that we're on the right track. And we are. As they swoop down to sit on our shoulders, our birds are singing of the correct shoe being on the foot of the true bride.

We're on the correct path because at last our true feminine, our container of uncompromised intuition, feelings, and creative potential is moving toward the ultimate union with the masculine's know-how, courage, and energy. Analyst Marilyn Matthews describes this inner pair this way: "Each brings along a sense of connection to the Self, an intrinsic sense of self-esteem and self-worth. Neither of them is affected by external appearances; each sees the reality of the other."

Final Sacrifice

As it becomes apparent that Cinderella is the true bride, the stepmother and sisters turn pale with outrage. In this they exhibit a symptom of depression, the fourth stage in the grieving process. This goes for us, too. At this point our stepsister ego knows the truth, but that doesn't stop us from still feeling some pain.

Bud and I moved to a new house the September before my fiftieth birthday, and while packing up I came across a photograph of me in my late twenties. Nostalgia for my youthful self welled up again, and I felt as though I'd run across the photo of a departed loved one. I even carried the picture around with me for a few days in hopes that by acknowledging my distress, it would fade away, as grief does when allowed to be aired. And my hunch was correct. My depression was short-lived.

This low state lasts only a short while in we who have allowed Cinderella's story to point the way to authentic appearance, because the one-sided nature of the stepmother and stepsisters are soon transmuted by the love between Cinderella and the prince. For, when the couple is free to marry, balance is returned to the family—that same state of equilibrium between the authentic feminine and masculine that was present before the good mother died and the father married the stepmother.

Finally, the stepsisters submit to the situation, which completes the last stage in the grieving process. Instead of trying to hold on to their old position as the only parlor sitters in the family, when time approaches for the royal wedding they come to Cinderella and want to get into her favor. With this acknowledgement of and acquiescence to her position as the true bride, they allow the old order to die away peacefully.

The subsequent action might surprise we who are unfamiliar with the allegorical nature of fairy tales. Mere mortals might play tit-for-tat with the stepsisters, either bursting into laughter at the very idea of honoring their request to remain with Cinderella or ordering them out of their sight, if not worse. But not Cinderella, whose birds sit on her shoulder and make her both wise and farsighted.

And it's the same with us if we but allow the story to progress in our lives. The birds know that Cinderella needs the parlor-sitting sisters who love pretty clothes and being out in public. And so do we, for they represent getting dressed up, going places, and experiencing things. Without the stepsisters, we might remain forever in the comfort of our internal castles—the place of daydreams and unfulfilled promise—never venturing forth to partake of what life has to offer. Thus, we would fail to contribute our midlife's work back to the world.

Our love of beautiful adornment hasn't been at the root of the parlor-related complex all these years anyway. It was our *false* notions about our appearance that caused the misery. Goodness knows, as we move into our upcoming decades we want to make ourselves beautiful, just as the Goddess does. What must be plucked from the stepsisters is their limited ability to recognize only *inauthentic* beauty.

Being blinded to the superficialities of the false persona—literally being rendered unaware of the attraction of youth and elitism—enables us to take the stepsisters' eye for beauty and turn it inward so that we behold the loveliness of the Self, both in us and in others. This is similar to Native American legend of how a mouse became an eagle. First, he was blinded on one side, then on the other. Then, with his former ability to see the superficialities of his small environment and fears gone, he was taken up into the sky where he merged with the eagle. For the same reason, prophets and oracles of old were either blind from birth or blinded at some point by the deities. Being blind made them wise because it forced them to turn to their inner vision for insight.

I often wake up in the middle of the night and feel the urge to go outside and just sit, especially when I'm up at the cabin. It's amazing how much better I perceive what's going on around me with the porch light off. In the dark, I hear the rich volume of crickets, owls, and scurrying animals. If I turn the light on, I mute their sound, because turning on the light separates me from being at one with the larger environment.

So, we needn't fear that blinding our egos to the glaring and glittery light of society's fixation on youth and wounded power will cripple us. Just the opposite—it's the Dark Mother who would have us slice off our toe and heel. Jungian analyst James Hollis claims in *The Middle Passage,* "As long as we remain primarily identified with the outer, objective world, we will be estranged from our subjective reality," and once we are estranged from subjective reality, we lose touch with the Self. Instead of estranging us, blinding our stepsisters enables us see ourselves and everyone else for who we and they truly are for the first time in our lives.

It's important to note that, on the way to the ceremony, each sister was only half-blinded and the sacrifice was completed after the royal wedding. For until the sacred nuptials are celebrated, the feminine and the masculine remain only half complete.

Although her primary realm is the unconscious, Cinderella must move into the conscious world as Queen, just as Persephone moved between Hades' underworld and Demeter's earth. The blinding that takes place before the wedding assures that the Cinderella in us will remain blind to the distraction of commercial beauty and society's fear of aging as she moves in and out of our consciousness.

The post-nuptial blinding helps strengthen the animus by raising his awareness of our inner knowledge, our intuition, even higher. We don't want him to get snared by the outer world, for he, too, must be able to travel both worlds. How else could he impregnate our soul with spirit so that we can continue to grow and walk in authentic beauty as we age if he isn't able to visit and unite with the queen of our innermost Self?

The Royal Wedding

The *hieros gamos,* or royal wedding, is as old as mythology and as universal as love. It's the sacred bonding of Mother Earth and Father Sky, Hera and Zeus, Shakti and Shiva, Christ and the Church—the union of feminine soul and masculine spirit. So, when the daughter of our true mother unites with the son of our good king, they do so in full partnership. Neither principle is paramount, because both are equally necessary.

And, because of their heroic trials and tribulations, they are mature in their own talents and powers. Being neither needy nor dependent, they are free of competition and the desire to coopt each other. They dance like two snakes in moonlit ecstasy of primal union—coming together and writhing, separating and going a distance by themselves, coming together again, and again separating—two beings who feel nothing more or less than the simple, glorious fullness of both themselves and the other simultaneously.

The cathedral wherein the royal marriage takes place is the physical symbol of their union. Thus, we honor and renew the marriage of soul and spirit each time we adorn our bodies—our personal temples—authentically. Inasmuch as we respect a cathedral for its sacredness, we refrain from desecrating it or rendering it incapable of housing the sacred. And, as with an altar in the woods, we understand that although it is sacred, it is merely the place of worship, not that which *is* worshipped.

Vows

By now you're fully aware that your desire for adornment is as natural as breathing, and that the issue isn't *what* you do to your body but *why* you choose to remake, redefine, and reshape it. As your king and queen unite in their holy marriage, you, too, make vows that concern how you will express and honor your Self. Not unexpectedly, there are seven vows that strengthen the royal marriage.

First Vow ⌐ *I will never forget that anyone selling a product or service, whether it be lipstick or liposuction, is out to make money.*
I don't care if the person is a licensed plastic surgeon, a celebrity on an infomercial, or the woman behind the cosmetic counter—each is there first and foremost to turn a profit. I'm not implying that they're all out to fleece you. I'm saying that what you hear from them is a sales pitch—a script that's been carefully crafted to shed the best possible light on their product.

Skin care specialists won't tell you outright that their creams will keep you from aging, but they'll come pretty darn close. Weight reduction counselors won't tell you directly that your self-esteem will rise a point with each pound shed, but that's the impression you'll get. And, yes, scientists and chemists work to develop cosmetics as advertised, but that doesn't mean that the products are all that good. The fact is, *all* creams, whether you buy them from Thrifty Drug Store or Neiman-Marcus, are developed by chemists. So when it comes to product claims, weigh the information against the profit motive and what you know about the fears inherent in the appearance complex, and choose wisely.

Second Vow ⌐ *I promise to ask questions.*
We've had the whammies put on us by the medical and beauty professions, leaving us to believe that they, like the gods, know all. But there's no

need for this "holier than thou" attitude from dermatologists, plastic surgeons, or anyone else who works on your body. Credible practitioners welcome questions, supply clear answers, and give lists of previous patients or clients whom you can call for a reference. It's your right as a consumer and your responsibility as the caretaker of your body to ask questions and demand satisfactory answers.

Furthermore, don't be seduced by a list of credentials following anyone's name. Questionable professional certificates, degrees, and memberships abound. Before someone works on you, research his or her background. You owe it to yourself. I sometimes think we're more concerned with the certification of our auto mechanics and veterinarians than we are with those who work on our bodies.

For goodness sake, don't be afraid to ask hard and direct questions about beauty products in terms of what you can expect from them, their ingredients, and any problems that might occur from their use. If you don't get the answers you seek, don't buy. And don't be afraid to shop around, either. No, you don't have to buy all your creams from one line, despite what you're told. Don't be intimidated into purchasing more than you really want. And, don't think for one minute that you can't return a skin-care or cosmetic product. You can, even if it's been opened and used.

Finally, understand full well that cosmetic surgery is full-blown surgery. The risks you take and the physical and psychic pain you incur are the same whether you're having your appendix out or a tummy tuck. So, before you indulge, weigh your parlor ego against your heart. As a litmus test, before you sign on the dotted line, consider whether or not you would subject your child or pet to the same surgery that you ask your body to endure.

Third Vow — *I understand that no amount of makeup, fine clothes, plastic surgery, dieting, or trips to a spa can shore up flailing self-esteem.*
It should be clear by now that just as Charlie the Tuna can't buy good taste,

we can't buy and wear good mental health. To be sure, there *is* a correlation between looking good and feeling good. Toward the end of a lengthy illness, my grandmother called the doctor and asked if she might go out long enough to visit the beauty parlor. Without hesitation he said, "This is the best news I've had all day. If you're wanting to get your hair done, you're on the road to recovery." Similarly, the old story about the woman who buys a new hat after a fight with her husband contains more armchair psychology than maybe we'd like to admit. We've all taken our wounded feelings to the mall and soothed them with a new cheek gloss or a new outfit (maybe even several).

But while nothing can create good feelings better in the short run than making ourselves look better, that's the extent a makeover or a new hair color can do. We can't sustain ourselves by remaking our appearance over the long haul if there isn't already a positive feeling of Self there to begin with. Beauty aids aren't medicine. They're barometers that register our inner condition, but they don't cure it.

What can we expect in the way of self-esteem when we decorate and remake our bodies? If a woman is *truly* unhappy with a *single* aspect of her appearance, such as a large nose, remaking it can improve her self-image. Thirty-eight-year-old Margaret's breasts were so small that she couldn't find bras in her size; after thinking it over carefully, she got implants. Fortunately, she's among those who haven't had medical repercussions, and ten years later she still feels great about her size 34C and has a grand time wearing sweaters. *But* she has no desire or need for more cosmetic surgery.

Fourth Vow ~ *I will remember that regardless of what is said by whom, nothing I can buy and little that I do can reduce the signs of aging over the long haul.*

The quality and texture of your skin has far more to do with your genes than anything you could ever rub on it. If you want to know how your skin will age, don't look into one of those fancy computer screens at a department store makeup counter, just look at your parents, grandparents, aunts, and uncles. In the long run, nothing can alter the quality and texture of your skin other than abstaining from sun, tobacco, and alcohol.

Still, for some of us, pampering our skin with $50-a-jar cream is a little comfort we extend to our otherwise over-stressed bodies. As my friend, Sally, put it, "It beats spending the same amount of money for a therapist to help me reduce stress. I'd rather spend it on a little luxury for myself."

I've heard this logic from more women than Sally. We feel that we work hard and have earned a few dollars to spend on ourselves. Sitting at an elegant counter and having a lovely-looking young woman sell us jars of cream is a treat. So is opening those exquisite little bottles each night and rubbing on the lotion. But let's realize when we spring for those jars that living out this fantasy of the pampered woman is just that, a fantasy. There's no harm in it, per se. In fact, the five minutes of pampering each night may even be good for us *if* we really do it as a treat for ourselves—a treat with no strings attached.

When it comes to applying color to our bodies, the danger lurks when we think that we aren't worthy without it. But applying color is Self-enhancing once we align with the royal pair. After the wedding a new shade of lipstick that rings true with our Self can send us soaring in less time and for less money than almost anything I can think of.

It's the same with diets and exercise. The harm or good depends on *why* we diet and exercise. We are a culture who latched on to the Duchess of Windsor's quip that "a woman can never be too rich or too thin" as a social mandate. However, adhering to this adage isn't for everybody.

Contrary to popular belief, the health risks of being overweight are far less severe than those of overdieting. Medical researchers claim that high blood pressure, heart attack, stroke, and diabetes, become problematic *only* when we weigh at least 35 percent more than our optimum weight. But many women who diet strenuously are nowhere near the optimum weight for their bone structures and heights, much less being 35 percent over it.

Yet, here's the rub. As we age into our mid-years, our natural body changes ready us for different physical needs, and excessive weight loss can impair the process. The pear-shaped body, so despised by middle-aged and older women, actually reduces the risk of heart attacks, because those unwanted cells in our hips and thighs store fat away from delicate organs and arteries in our upper body. They also store essential vitamins and minerals that stave off osteoporosis and other conditions that plague older women.

In addition, maintaining an abnormally low weight depletes us, both emotionally and physically. This becomes an especially crucial issue when menopausal hormonal changes already may be playing havoc with us. Diets can leave us feeling extra tired and irritable as well as unnecessarily depressed. Yet even if we put menopause aside, it's a proven fact that hungry bodies don't feel good, and the effects of yo-yo dieting play cat and mouse with even the healthiest self-esteem. On one hand we may believe that maintaining that size eight we wore in college is paramount to feeling worthy as we pass forty; but on the other, we may do more to undermine our self-esteem than if we allow ourselves to go up a size or two.

When it comes to exercise and our overall well-being, the payoffs may be more forthcoming. A well-developed exercise program not only trims and reshapes the body but decreases our chances of heart attacks, osteoporosis, certain types of arthritis, and other conditions that beset us in our middle and later years. And exercise's most valuable outcome is the increase in our body's level of endorphins—those valuable, natural chemicals that produce emotional highs. Maintaining a steady supply of endorphins through regular exercise can do more for our mental health and bodies during menopause and beyond than all the plastic surgery and cosmetics money can buy.

But again, to determine if our exercise is linked in any way to the false parlor, we need to analyze *why* we exercise and *what* we believe we're getting from it, not just whether we do it or not. I'm personally troubled by the term *hard body* in that I perceive the persona associated with it as a tough little cookie who's all brawn and bravado with no soul—the movie roles often played by Jamie Lee Curtis and the like. Believe me, this form of female strength is the antithesis of soul-building, for the aggressiveness and machismo we develop from extreme outer body work in no way substitutes for authentic feminine power.

If used correctly, however, exercise is a great way to reclaim dominion over our bodies. Many midlife women report new feelings of power as they develop muscles *along with* tackling the inner journey. The combination allows them to "muscle" back control over their bodies, thus contributing to a healthier overall self-concept. In this regard, I'm elated at the rise in popularity of t'ai chi, yoga, and dance therapy, that combine the spiritual with the physical.

Fifth Vow — *I will be honest with myself and others about my appearance.* Dishonesty about what we do to our bodies and why we do it is a sure sign that we're still tied to the false parlor—a signal that our makeup, face-lift, or weight reduction program is more than a minor correction or an outlet for creativity. To this end, let's examine five questions we want to ask ourselves before making any substantial change.

- Will I be comfortable discussing the change openly with others, or will I feel the need to hide or misrepresent what I'm about to do?
- Do I accept the fact that the change will likely not add to my long-term feelings of well-being, or do I cling to the hope that it will shore up my life in some way?
- Do I understand that I am equally valuable with or without the change, or do I expect that the change will result in more friends or more love and attention from my significant other?

- Does my desire for change come from my Self, or is it a reaction to a *should?*
- Do I really want and need the change, or am I just restless and wanting to do something different to myself?

The answer *yes* to the second half of any of these questions is a red flag—a warning that your expected satisfaction with the outcome of the change will elude you. If your answer is *no* to the last part of each question, chances are you may be operating from your Self.

Sixth Vow — *I will remember that the fashion industry can and will serve me rather than the other way around.*
It's true. Although we may not have believed it before we developed an authentic appearance, the fashion industry isn't a powerful god. It merely provides our clothes and cosmetics—nothing more, nothing less. As such, it *will* respond to the demands of middle-aged women who wish to age positively, because to stay in business the designers, retailers, fashion magazines, and cosmetic companies must sell us their products. We who are in our forties, fifties, and sixties have more money to spend on clothing and grooming products than any other age group. Let's use our financial power to get what we want.

Knowing that you can vote for how you want to be treated with your dollars, let the buyers at your local department stores know that you don't want fashions that make you look like a teenager. Write to the editors of your favorite magazines and complain about being shown clothes on models who are one-third your age. Years ago I dropped my subscription to *Lear's* for that very reason—they failed to answer my question about their choice of models, so I chose to keep my money. Call the hands of cosmetic consultants and skin care specialists when they begin to speak to you about needing to look younger. They'll soon get the message that you look the age you are, and that's that. Then they will gladly provide the products and services you want sans the guilt trip.

Even though the fashion and beauty industries have a long way to go in acknowledging our right to an authentic appearance, I'm beginning to see a slight falling away of the old mindset. For example, a few of the catalogs I receive, such as Land's End, show a few older models. This first step in the right direction is an indication that change *can* take place. But the industry won't go the full distance without us pushing it along with our demands.

Seventh Vow — *I promise to continue to age positively.*
We know from experience that Cinderella and the prince really can't ride off on a horse and live happily ever after without a great deal of daily work to keep their relationship strong. So we can't expect that we will fulfill the promise of our second half without conscious and constant attention to positive aging. The following are but a few suggestions that will assure that your royal marriage will grow over the years to come. Several were gleaned from groups who support an authentic appearance, such as the San Francisco–based About-Face. Others come from my experiences with women who've aged in beauty and wisdom.

- Stop talking negatively about your weight, flab, and wrinkles, especially in front of young, impressionable girls. This will help curb the spread of inauthentic appearance more than any single thing I can think of.
- Keep a list of older women whom you admire for what they do rather than merely how they look. Update it regularly and refer to it often. You might even compare lists with your friends.
- Continue to reward yourself for jobs well done by buying jewelry. This arsenal of personal power symbols will take you further into your later years than all the financial and career planning you can do.
- Talk, talk, talk with friends, associates, and significant others about authentic appearance and positive aging. The more we talk about it,

the more we, and they, do it. This raises everyone up to new heights and takes the invisibility and negativity out of the aging process.

- Support other women in their quest for authentic aging. Part of what keeps us in the parlor is feeling that we are alone. And that's how we stay—alone—unless we join together and enlighten each other. I have a poster in my office put out by the American Association of University Women that says, "We're changing the world *one woman at a time*." And that's how we will change society's attitude about our aging bodies—one woman at a time—when we reach other women in a one-on-one basis.

To Love and to Honor

I teach a psychology course on the self in society. One of the most difficult concepts to get across to my students is that of individuation. These young folks look at middle adulthood as a time when they'll have it all in terms of living the way they want to—that they will be responsible to no one except themselves. They like that—being able to do whatever they want but not having to worry about anything or anyone getting in their way. To put my response to their interpretation of individuation in their vernacular, "Wrong!" Individuation doesn't mean anything goes.

Since our bodies are *wakan* (sacred feminine) and the spirit is borne by *susquan* (sacred masculine), how we relate to them and the decisions we make about them can either defile or glorify their holy nature. What we do to our physical bodies, the looks we create, and the roles we play out via our appearance, particularly as we age, all matter on the metaphysical plane. That we've been entrusted with our bodies, therefore, is no small gift—it's *awesome*.

We must, therefore, take full responsibility for our bodies—what we put into our bodies, what we do to our bodies, and what we expect from them—from the perspective of their sacredness. Are the choices we've made up until now good choices? If not, can we correct them? How and when? Be assured, this is no cause to lash out at yourself for what might seem to have been a mistake. Remember that whatever was done, was done. Simple as that. Inasmuch as the royal couple didn't banish or kill the stepsisters, they aren't harsh judges, and they have no room in their realm for guilt. So neither do we.

Before we make any major decisions about remaking or radically altering our bodies, it's a good idea to go to our sacred place, sit down, and ask our inner wisewoman what *she* thinks. If, instead of letting her answer, you begin to justify or argue why you need the change, better think it through again. She's probably not telling you what you want to hear. But if the final answer from your heart-of-hearts is clear, affirming, and loving, a change may be in order.

As I began writing this chapter I got a call from a friend who wanted to lose twenty-five pounds but didn't know whether that might be a reasonable amount for her body. Since I'm no expert on diets and am unqualified to give her such advice, I suggested that she ask her body what it thought was a fair amount to lose. When she did, she came to the conclusion that fifteen pounds would do, rather than twenty-five.

When it comes to the responsibility we have toward others, we may have to do more than have a talk with our Self. As healing requires that we rerecord those negative tapes that play constantly in our heads, I suggest you become conscious of the thoughts you have about other women, particularly midlife and older women, as you go about your daily tasks. Once you analyze what you've been programmed to think about others in light of what you know about the good mother and true king residing in *all* of us, those hateful tapes become noxious, and you'll shut them down. Too, as you blind your ego's eyes to false parlor beauty and inauthenticity loses its grip on your appearance, you'll naturally lighten up on other women. As you remove yourself from the appearance hot seat, so shall you remove others (surely there's a golden rule in there somewhere!).

The bottom line, of course, is that we are *all* good and worthy women—not just some of us. Once this idea sinks in, we no longer want to remain separate from others, because women of all stages, ages, and circumstances have a lot to contribute to us, and we to them. Finally, it becomes unthinkable that we would ever have excluded anyone—especially on account of her age and how she looked.

The next step beyond eliminating the negative, obviously, is to develop the positive—to learn to recognize beauty in other women. And I guarantee you'll find it.

As you look around with your inner eye, you'll see beautiful young girls on the streets of South-Central Los Angeles, middle-aged women in markets and malls on the plains of Kansas, and well-appointed crones walking down Fifth Avenue. You'll find silver-haired wisewomen in nursing homes everywhere. And the genuinely beautiful women you see will make the slick photographs in *People, Vogue,* and *W* banal by comparison.

We who have united with our Self must also accept a great deal of responsibility because we are connected to *all* things. As such, we are 100 percent responsible for maintaining and adorning our bodies in such a way as to not disturb the very delicate ecosystem we live in.

This is a tall order and may sound radically New Age. But it's as old as the Kentucky hills. When the southwestern Native Americans talk of walking in beauty they speak of more, by far, than looking good. It's the philosophy that each of us is connected to all things, and that all things are connected to us. As such, we are to honor the Divine spirit in everything. And when we honor this all-in-all spirit, we walk in authentic beauty.

And truly, as we move deeper into our Selves, we come to know on a plane that is far from our conscious understanding that indeed we *are* connected. Once we feel this connectedness, we can never again conceive of ourselves as separate beings—independent yes, but not separate. We have a great and grave responsibility to make conscientious decisions about what we wear and the products we use—ones that will ensure to the best of our abilities that everything in nature is as cared for as possible.

I cannot tell you what choices to make. These are up to you. You may become sensitive to animal testing and choose to buy beauty products that aren't tested on laboratory animals. I and many other women no longer wear animal furs. I have several friends who refuse to buy clothing made in China and other countries that have poor human rights records. The list of possibilities is endless because of the hundreds of dangerous and inhumane activities that permeate the making of our clothing and beauty products.

By going inside and conferring with the good Mother, you'll come to your own conclusions. And then it becomes easier than you might think to act on your newly awakened convictions.

In Full Bloom

We began with the story of Narcissus, the ill-fated youth who loved nothing but his own reflection and was turned into a small white flower, rimmed in pale red. We finish our journey as roses, the variety known as Double-Delight, which begin as does the narcissus with small white petals tinged with red-pink. But at full maturity, they are lush with outer petals of rich crimson that melt into pure white near the stem, while their center petals are as yellow as the king's sun. Like them, our ripe beauty mirrors these colors of the loving mother and the powerful king.

As middle-aged women adorned in the royal splendor of authenticity, we're enabled to resolve conflicts with love in our hearts for all concerned. We know when to give our tired bodies a rest, allow some slack when we're too hard on ourselves, rise above pettiness, and choose far-ranging rather than short-term payoffs. We have the dignity to congratulate ourselves for jobs well done and congratulate others for the same. We consider the good of all creation in our decisions. We have the courage to back down when we're wrong and fight to the bitter end for that which we feel in our heart-of-hearts is right. We acknowledge the authentic beauty in our daughters, sisters, mothers, and grandmothers.

Above all we contain within us a royal child who is waiting to be born. Your royal child is the fruit of your creativity, whether it be manifest in your daily routine or putting the finishing touches on your life's greatest accomplishment to date. For these activities are but one in the same— a celebration of your beautiful and authentic Self.

As you walk on mother earth, celebrate under father sky, create the royal child day in and day out, and age positively in your coming years, take the essence of a traditional Navajo blessing with you:

> *May you walk with beauty before you*
> *May you walk with beauty behind you*
> *May you walk with beauty below you*
> *May you walk with beauty above you*
> *May beauty encircle you*
> *May beauty restore you.*

⁓ Acknowledgments

As I look through my window this October morning, I'm filled with wonder at the variegated patchwork—a quilt of various sizes, colors, and configurations of leaves. This is what it took to make this book, a patch-work of people who contributed stories, time, interest, support, tears, laughter, and well-wishes so that my words could spring forth.

Because unraveling who contributed what could never be complete or all-inclusive, I hesitate. But in my gratitude, I'm willing to risk such sins of omission and commission.

Mother is my rock, my soul builder—a crone high priestess in the ancient sense. Daddy, who prizes education above all else, never bought into the notion that girls and women *couldn't* or *shouldn't;* thus I can and do. Granny, full of folk wisdom, tinged with a love for English literature, taught me about gardens and storytelling and being kind to the birds. Ma-Keg led me into Grimm's dark mythological forests and magical lands where the prince and princess lived. To these grandmothers I say, "Thank you for being who and what the child needed." I'm indebted to Herby, my maternal grandfather and his family for being spirit bearers. And, to my Celtic and Cherokee forebearers, I give honor and a place of recognition in my life.

My husband, Bud, is the lift beneath my wings, believing in me and my abilities long before I did. I couldn't have written without Maggie, our cocker spaniel, who sat at my feet and was my most constant companion as I wrote. I am grateful for the encouragement of my stepdaughter, Misha, whose bright voice is ever ready to cheer me through the rough spots in the road.

An adage says that we will have five good friends throughout our life-time, and I'm blessed with having four of the five thus far. Fran Carroll,

Mary K. Ericksen, Zelda Gilbert, and Jackie Shadko, my soulmates whose senses of humor, wisdom, soft shoulders, unfailing faith in this project, and personal generosity carried me further and longer than I can describe. To them I say, "Thanks for being there. I couldn't have done it without ya."

I would like to thank Woodbury University and President Paul Sago (retired) for financial assistance and the sabbatical that enabled my research and training in Jungian psychology. To my Woodbury colleagues who gave special support, I say a wholehearted thank you: Iris Addonisio, Joan Angeles, Carol Bishop, Ellen Campbell, Mary Collins, Doug Cremer, Shally Dhiman, Maureen Ettinger, Geraldine Forbes, Hoda Meisamy, Brad Monsma, Lou Naidorf, Marvin Richman, Elisabeth Sandberg, Noelle Sharp, Rosalie Utterbach, and Katherine Richards and her library staff.

Other friends to whom I am grateful are Paul Gilbert, Ross and Anne Sonne, Ashley Carroll, Kay Mouradian, Rodka Donnell, Lynn Creighton, Nancy Moore, and Mike Stephans.

Then there are those who helped hone my writing skills and/or the manuscript: Jean-Noel Bassior, Regula Noetzli, and Ken Atchity. I'm grateful to the women who participated in my research, attended my seminars and/or shared their stories with me. I'm especially indebted to Mary Jane Ryan and everyone at Conari Press for giving me the opportunity to sing my midlife song. I thank those at the Jung Institutes in Los Angeles, San Francisco, and Küsnacht (Switzerland), in particular Kathrin Asper and Ruth Ammann for providing the framework for understanding the feminine psyche through fairy tales.

Finally, I owe all that I am and, thus, all that I say to the Alpha and the Omega: Great Spirit.

➤ Bibliography

Allen, Paula Gunn. *Spider Woman's Granddaughters*. Boston: Beacon Press, 1989.

_____. *The Sacred Hoop*. Boston: Beacon Press, 1992.

Ammann, Ruth. "Grandmothers, Mothers & Daughters." Lectures, C. G. Jung Institute, Küsnacht, Switzerland (January 9–10, 1995).

_____. "The Verdant Ones: Figures of Green Men and Green Women." Lecture, C. G. Jung Institute, San Francisco (September 29, 1995).

_____. "The House and Garden in Fairy Tales." workshop, C. G. Jung Institute, San Francisco (October 1, 1995).

Andersen, Hans Christian, "The Emperor's New Clothes" in *It's Perfectly True*. Paul Leyssac (trans.). New York: Harcourt, Brace & World, Inc., 1966.

Anderson, Lorraine, ed. *Sisters of the Earth: Women's Prose and Poetry About Nature*. New York: Vintage Books, 1991.

Andrews, Ted. *Animal-Speak: The Spiritual & Magical Powers of Creatures Great & Small*. St. Paul: Llewellyn Publications, 1995.

Aquinas, Thomas, in Umberto Eco, *Art and Beauty in the Middle Ages*. New Haven: Yale University Press, 1986, 70.

Asper, Kathrin. *The Abandoned Child Within: On Losing and Regaining Self Worth*. New York: Fromm International, 1993.

_____. "The Search for Identity in Fairy Tales." Lectures, C. G. Jung Institute, Küsnacht, Switzerland (January 5–6, 1995).

Atkinson, Holly. *Women and Fatigue*. New York: Putnam, 1985.

Baker, Nancy C. *The Beauty Trap*. New York: Franklin Watts, 1984.

Bancroft, Anne. *Weavers of Wisdom: Women Mystics of the Twentieth Century*. Hammondsworth, England: Arkana, 1989.

Banner, Lois. *American Beauty*. University of Chicago Press: Chicago, 1984.

Barthel, Diane. *Putting on Appearances: Gender and Advertising*. Philadelphia: Temple University Press, 1988.

Beck, Peggy, Anna Lee Walters, and Nia Francisco. *The Sacred: Ways of Knowledge, Sources of Life* (redesigned ed.). Tsaile, AZ: Navaho Community College Press, 1995.

Belenky, Mary Field, Blythe McVicker Clinchy, Nancy Rule Goldberger, and Jill Mattuck Tarule. *Women's Way of Knowing*. New York: Basic Books, 1986.

Bernard, Jean. "The Hand and the Mind." *Parabola* X:3 (Fall 1993): 14–17.

Biedermann, Hans. *Dictionary of Symbolism: Cultural Icons & The Meanings Behind Them*. James Hulbert (trans.). New York: Meridian, 1994.

Bielese, Megan. "The Old Ones Give You Life." *Parabola* V:1 (Winter 1990): 39–46.

Black Elk, Wallace, and William S. Lyon. *Black Elk: The Sacred Ways of a Lakota*. San Francisco: Harper & Row, 1990.

Blass, Bill, in Etta Froio's "New York's Bad Boys," *W.* (December 1993),121.

Blyth, R. H., in F. Franck, "Living Ancestors." *Parabola* V:5 (1980): 25–26.

Bolen, Jean Shinoda. *Crossing to Avalon*. San Francisco: Harper, 1994.

_____. "When the Ground Gives Way: Earth-Shaking Events and the Meaning of Life." workshop, C. G. Jung Institute, San Francisco (October 14, 1995).

Bond, D. Stephenson. *Living Myth*. Boston: Shambhala, 1993.

Bradshaw, John. *Healing the Shame That Binds You*. Deerfield Beach, Fla.: Health Communications, 1988.

Brandon, Nathaniel. *Honoring the Self*. Los Angeles: J. P. Tarcher, 1983.

Brothers, Dr. Joyce. "Beauty May Lead to a Beastly Life." *Los Angeles Times* (May 17, 1990).

_____. "Beauty Doesn't Ensure Happiness." *Los Angeles Times* (June 15, 1993).

_____. "Mirror, Mirror: Are Looks Really Important?" *Los Angeles Times* (June 15, 1993).

Brown, Joseph Epes. *The Spiritual Legacy of the American Indian*. New York: Crossroads, 1986.

Brownmiller, Susan. *Femininity*. New York: Linden Press, 1984.

Burckhardt, Jacob. *The Civilization of the Renaissance in Italy*. New York: The Modern Library, 1954.

Burckhart, Titus. "The Return of Ulysses." *Parabola* III:4 (1978): 16–20.

Campbell, Joseph. *The Masks of God: Primitive Mythology*. New York: Penguin, 1969.

_____. *Myths to Live By*. New York: Penguin, 1972.

_____. "Joseph Campbell on the Great Goddess." *Parabola* V:4 (1980): 74–85.

Cassier, Ernst. *The Individual and the Cosmos in Renaissance Philosophy*. Philadelphia: University of Pennsylvania Press, 1963.

Cheney, Sheldon. *Men Who Have Walked With God*. New York: Alfred A. Knopf, 1956.

Chernin, Kim. *The Hungry Self*. New York: Times Books, 1985.

Cirlot, J. E. *A Dictionary of Symbols*. Jack Sage (trans.). New York: Philosophical Library, 1983.

Clance, Dr. Pauline Rose. *The Impostor Phenomenon*. Atlanta: Peachtree Publishers, 1985.

Clark, Miles. *Every Day I Have a Journey*. New York: Harper & Row, 1976.

Complete Grimm's Fairy Tales. New York: Random House, 1972.

Corriere, Richard, and Joseph Hart. *Psychological Fitness*. New York: Harcourt Brace Jovanovich, 1979.

Critchlow, Keith. "The Soul as Sphere and Androgyne." *Parabola* III:4 (Fall 1974): 34–40.

Damascius, *Epitaph*. (Greek Anthology. Bk. vii, epig. 533) in Burton Stevenson, *The Home Book of Quotations*. New York: Dodd, Mead & Company, 1967, 175.

"Dateline." *Los Angeles Times* (June 26, 1992).

Davis, Fred. *Fashion, Culture, and Identity*. Chicago: University of Chicago Press, 1992.

Douglas, Claire. *The Woman in the Mirror*. Boston: Sigo, 1990.

Douglas, Mary. *Natural Symbols*. New York: Pantheon Books, 1970.

Doyle, Thomas B. "Survival of the Fittest." *American Demographics* (May 1989): 38–41.

Dunne, John S. *The Way of All the Earth*. New York: Macmillan, 1972.

Eaton, Evelyn. *I Send a Voice*. Wheaton, IL: Theosophical Publishing House, 1978.

Eco, Umberto. *Art and Beauty in the Middle Ages*. New Haven: Yale University Press, 1986.

Eisler, Riane. *The Chalice & the Blade*. San Francisco: HarperSanFrancisco, 1987.

"Elders and Guides: A Conversation with Joseph Campbell." *Parabola* V:1 (1980): 57–65.

Eliot, Alexander. *The Universal Myths: Heroes, Tricksters and Others*. New York: Meridian, 1990.

Erdoes, Richard, and Alfonso Ortiz. *American Indian Myths and Legends*. New York: Pantheon Books, 1984.

Estés, Clarissa Pinkola. *Women Who Run With the Wolves*. New York: Ballantine Books, 1993.

Fallon, April E., and Paul Rozin. "Sex Differences in Perceptions of Desirable Body Shape." *Journal of Abnormal Psychology* 94:1 (1985): 102–105.

Finley, John M. *Considering Plastic Surgery?* Gretna: Pelican, 1991.

Foster, Steven, and Meredith Little. *The Roaring of the Sacred River*. New York: Prentice-Hall, 1989.

Franck, Frederick. "Living Ancestors." *Parabola* V:5 (1980): 26.

Freedman, Rita. *Beauty Bound*. Lexington, Mass.: Lexington Books, 1986.

Frymer-Kensky, Tikva. *In the Wake of the Goddess:Women, Culture, and the Biblical Transformation of Pagan Myth*. New York: The Free Press, 1992.

Gadon, Elinor W. *The Once & Future Goddess*. San Francisco: Harper & Row, 1989.

Gaudoin, Tina. "Makeup." *Harper's Bazaar* (October 1992): 325–398.

Gergen, Kenneth J. *The Saturated Self*. New York: Basic Books, 1991.

Graves, Robert. *The Greek Myths: 1*. Middlesex, England: Penguin, 1955.

Goffman, Erving. *The Presentation of Self in Everyday Life*. Garden City, NY: Doubleday, 1959.

Grimm, Jacob, and Wilhelm Grimm. *Selected Tales*. David Luke (trans.). London: Penguin Books, 1982.

Haederele, Michael. "Spirited Away: Native American Rituals Are Trendy. But Is This Homage or Another Rip-off?" *Los Angeles Times* (March 31, 1994).

Hamel, Ruth. "Raging Against Aging." *American Demographics* (March 1990): 42–45.

Hanna, Barbara. *Encounters With the Soul: Active Imagination as Developed by C. G. Jung*. Santa Monica, CA: Sigo Press, 1981.

Hirshfield, Jane, ed. *Women in Praise of the Sacred*. New York: HarperCollins, 1994.

Hitze, Franz. *Geburtenrückgang und Sozialreform*. Mönchengladbach: Volksverien, 1917, 93.

Hochswender, Woody. "Appearance at Work." *Vogue* (October 1991).

Hollis, James. *The Middle Passage: From Misery to Meaning in Midlife*. Toronto: Inner City Books, 1993.

_____. *Under Saturn's Shadow: The Wounding and Healing of Men*. Toronto: Inner City Books, 1994.

Homer. *The Odyssey of Homer*. Richmond Lattimore (trans.). New York: Harper & Row, 1965.

Hopcke, Robert H. *Persona*. Boston: Shambhala, 1995.

Howels, William. *The Heathens: Primitive Man and His Religion*. Garden City, NY: Doubleday and Company, 1948.

Hutchinson, Marcia Germaine. *Transforming Body Image*. Freedom, CA: Crossing Press, 1992.

Jeffers, Susan. *Feel the Fear and Do It Anyway*. New York: Fawcett Columbine, 1987.

Johnson, Robert A. *Inner Work*. San Francisco: HarperSanFrancisco, 1986.

_____. *She* (rev. ed.). New York: Harper Perennial, 1989.

Jongeward, David. *Weaver of Worlds*. Rochester, NY: Destiny Books, 1990.

Jung, Carl G. *The Undiscovered Self*. R. F. C. Hull (trans.). Boston: Little, Brown & Co., 1957.

_____. *Man and His Symbols*. Garden City, NY: Doubleday & Company, 1964.

Kaiser, Susan. *The Social Psychology of Dress* (2d ed.). New York: Macmillan, 1990.

Kamperidis, Lambros. "Surrounded by Water and Dying of Thirst." *Parabola* XVII:1 (Spring 1992): 12–17.

Keats, John. "Ode on a Grecian Urn." *The Works of John Keats*. Roslyn, NY: Black's Readers Service Company, 1951.

Kelsea, Maura. "Beyond the Stethoscope: A Nurse Practitioner Looks at Menopause and Midlife" in Dena Taylor and Amber Coverdale Sumerall (eds.), *Women of the 14th Moon*. Freedom, CA: Crossing Press, 1991, 274.

Kisley, Lorraine, "Focus." *Parabola* IV (Fall 1980): 3.

Kolodny, Annette. *The Land Before Her*. Chapel Hill: University of North Carolina Press, 1984.

Labarge, Margaret Wade. *A Small Sound of the Trumpet*. Boston: Beacon, 1986.

La Belle, Jenijoy. *Herself Beheld*. Ithaca, NY: Cornell University Press, 1988.

Langner, Lawrence. *The Importance of Wearing Clothes*. New York: Hastings House, 1959.

Larrington, Carolyne, ed. *Feminist Companion to Mythology*. London: Pandora Press, 1992.

Laver, James. *Costumes in Antiquity*. New York: Potter, 1964.

Leach, Maria, ed. *Funk and Wagnalls Standard Dictionary of Folklore, Mythology, and Legend*. San Francisco: Harper, 1972.

Leonard, Linda Schierse. *Meeting the Madwoman*. New York: Bantam Books, 1993.

Lerner, Harriet. "Harriet Lerner's Good Advice." *New Woman* (August 1996): 56.

Levi-Straus, Claude. *The Savage Mind*. Chicago: University of Chicago Press, 1966.

Louden, Jennifer. *The Woman's Comfort Book*. San Francisco: Harper, 1992.

Luhan, Mable Dodge, in L. Anderson (ed.), *Sisters of the Earth:Women's Prose and Poetry About Nature*. New York:Vintage Books, 1991, 97.

Luke, Helen M. "The Perennial Feminine." *Parabola* IV (Fall 1980): 10–23.

———. *Old Age: Journey into Simplicity*. New York: Parabola Books, 1987.

Lysne, Robin Heerens. *Dancing Up the Moon: A Woman's Guide to Creating Traditions that Bring Sacredness to Daily Life*. Berkeley: Conari Press, 1995.

Maslow, Abraham. *Motivation and Personality* (2d ed.). New York: Harper & Row, 1970.

Mason, Marilyn J. *Making Our Lives Our Own*. San Francisco: HarperSanFrancisco, 1991.

Matthews, Marilyn. "'The Snow Queen': An Interpretation" in M. Stein and L. Corbett (eds.), *Psyche's Stories*. 2 vols. Wilmette, IL: Chiron Publications, 1992, 88.

McKnight, Michael. "Elders and Guides: A Conversation with Joseph Campbell." *Parabola* I (1980): 57–67.

Medicine Eagle, Brooke. "Grandmother Wisdom: Lessons of the Moon-Pause Lodge." Audiotape. Guerneville, CA: Harmony Network.

Melamed, Elissa. *Mirror, Mirror: The Terror of Not Being Young*. New York: Linden Press/Simon and Schuster, 1983.

Melphmene Institute for Women's Health Research, The. *Bodywise Woman*. New York: Prentice Hall, 1990.

Merton, Thomas. *Love and Living*. New York: Farrar-Straus-Giroux, 1979.

Mitchell, Roy. *The Exile of the Soul*. John. L. Davenport (ed.). Buffalo, NY: Prometheus Books, 1983.

Moore, Thomas. *Care of the Soul*. New York: Harper Perennial, 1992.

Monaghan, Patricia. *The Book of Goddesses & Heroines*. St. Paul, MN: Llewellyn Publications, 1993.

Montagu, Ashley. *Man: His First Two Million Years*. New York: Dell Publishing, 1969.

Moreau, Catherine. "The Many-Sided Animus." Lectures, C. G. Jung Institute, Küsnacht, Switzerland (January 12–13, 1995).

Murdock, Maureen. *The Heroine's Journey: Woman's Quest for Wholeness*. Boston: Shambhala, 1990.

⸺⸺⸺. *The Hero's Daughter*. New York: Fawcett Columbine, 1994.

Native Peoples. 8:1 (Fall 1994): 36.

New Larousse Encyclopedia of Mythology. New York: Prometheus Press, 1968.

Norris, Kathleen. "A Glorious Robe." *Parabola* XIX:3 (August 1994): 45–48.

Nystrom, Paul. *The Economics of Fashion*. New York: Ronald Press Company, 1928.

Odermatt, Martin. "Guilt, Anxiety & Individuation." Lectures, C. G. Jung Institute, Küsnacht, Switzerland (January 12–13, 1995).

Padilla, Stan. *Chants and Prayers: A Native American Circle of Beauty*. Summertown, TN: The Book Publishing Company, 1995.

Paulus, Trina. *Hope for the Flowers*. New York: Paulist Press, 1972.

Peach, Emily. *Tarot for Tomorrow*. Irthlingborough, England: Woolnough Book-binding Limited, 1988.

Pipher, Mary. *Reviving Ophelia: Saving the Selves of Adolescent Girls*. New York: Ballantine Books, 1994.

Plato, *The Republic*. Bk. iii, sec. 402. Benjamin Jowlett, M.A. (trans.). New York: P. F. Collier & Son, 1901, 87.

Randolph, Laura B. "Oprah Opens Up About Her Weight, Her Wedding and Why She Withheld the Book." *Ebony* (October 1993): 130–137.

Rinse, Rip. "The Next Logical Step in Dressing." *Los Angeles Times* (November 10, 1994): E1.

Roderick, Timothy. *The Once Unknown Familiar*. St. Paul, MN: Llewellen Publications, 1994.

Rosenberg, Morris. *Conceiving the Self*. New York: Basic Books, 1979.

Rosenfeld, Megan. "The Story on Toys for Girls? They're Mostly About Boys." *Los Angeles Times* (January 4, 1996): E10.

Roth, Geneen. *When Food Is Love*. New York: Dutton, 1991.

Rountree, Cathleen. *On Women Turning 50*. San Francisco: Harper, 1993.

Russian Fairy Tales from the collections of Aleksandr Afanas'ev, Norbert Guterman (trans.). New York: Random House, 1973.

Salk, Jonas. *Survival of the Wisest*. New York: Harper & Row, 1973.

Sams, Jamie, and David Carson. *Medicine Cards: The Discovery of Power Through the Ways of Animals*. Santa Fe: Bear & Company, 1988.

Samuels, Mike. *Healing With the Mind's Eye*. New York: Summit Books, 1990.

Sanford, Linda Tschirhart, and Mary Ellen Donovan. *Women and Self-Esteem*. Garden City, NY: Anchor Press/Doubleday, 1984.

Schectman, Jacqueline. *The Step Mother in Fairytales*. Boston: Sigo Press, 1993.

Shakespeare, William. *The Tragedy of Macbeth* (revised). Eugene M. Waith (ed.). New Haven: Yale University Press, 1954.

Sheehy, Gail. *The Silent Passage*. New York: Random House, 1992.

Spenden, Herbert Joseph. *Songs of the Tewa* (2d ed.). Santa Fe, NM: Sunstone Press, 1993.

Stein, Diane. *Casting the Circle: A Woman's Book of Ritual*. Freedom, CA: Crossing Press, 1992.

Steinem, Gloria. *Revolution From Within*. Boston: Little, Brown & Co., 1992.

Stein, M., and L. Corbett, eds. *Psyche's Stories*, vol. I. Wilmette, IL: Chiron Publications, 1991.

_____. *Psyche's Stories*, vol. II. Wilmette, IL: Chiron Publications, 1992.

_____. *Psyche's Stories*, vol. III. Wilmette, IL: Chiron Publications, 1995.

Stevens, Anthony. *On Jung*. London: Routledge, 1990.

Stone, Christopher. *Re-Creating Your Self*. Portland: Metamorphous Press, 1988.

Storr, Anthony. *Solitude*. New York: Ballantine Books, 1988.

Taylor, Dena, and Amber Coverdale Sumerall, eds. *Women of the 14th Moon*. Freedom, CA: Crossing Press, 1991.

Taylor, Terry Lynn. *Guardians of Hope*. Tiburon, CA: H. J. Kramer Inc., 1992.

_____. *Creating With the Angels*. Tiburon, CA: H. J. Kramer Inc., 1993.

Tuana, Nancy. *Woman and the History of Philosophy*. Dallas: University of Texas, 1992.

Veblen, Thorstein. *The Theory of the Leisure Class*. New York: Macmillan, 1899.

Vlahos, Olivia. *Body: The Ultimate Symbol*. New York: J. B. Lippincott Company.

Vogue (April 1992).Reebok™ advertisements pp. 313–20.

von Franz, Marie-Louise. *The Feminine in Fairy Tales* (rev. ed). Boston: Shambhala, 1993.

_____. *Shadow and Evil in Fairy Tales* (rev. ed). Boston: Shambhala, 1995.

Walker, Barbara G. *The Woman's Encyclopedia of Myths and Secrets*. New York: HarperCollins, 1983.

_____. *The Crone: Woman of Age, Wisdom, and Power*. New York: HarperCollins, 1985.

_____. *The Woman's Dictionary of Symbols & Sacred Objects*. San Francisco: HarperSanFrancisco, 1988.

Wall, Steve. *Wisdom's Daughters*. New York: Harper Perennial, 1993.

_____. *Shadowcatchers*. New York: Harper Perennial, 1994.

Wolf, Naomi. *The Beauty Myth*. New York: William Morrow, 1991.

Wolff, Toni. "Structural Forms of the Feminine Psyche." Paul Watzlawik (trans.). Zurich: C. G. Jung Institute, 1992.

Woodman, Marion. *Conscious Femininity*. Toronto: Inner City Books, 1993.

_____. "The Stillness Shall Be the Dancing." Audiotape. College Station: Texas A&M University Press, 1994.

Woodman, Marion, and Elinor Dickson. *Dancing in the Flames: The Dark Goddess in the Transformation of Consciousness*. Boston: Shambhala, 1996.

Woolger, Jennifer Barker, and Roger J. Woolger. *The Goddess Within*. New York: Fawcett Columbine, 1989.

Yungblut, John R. *Discovering God Within*. Philadelphia: Westminister Press, 1979.

Zahner-Roloff, Lee. "'Snow White and Rose Red' Contained Opposites" in M. Stein and L. Corbett (eds.), *Psyche's Stories,* vol II. Wilmette, IL: Chiron Publications, 1992, 121.

~ Index

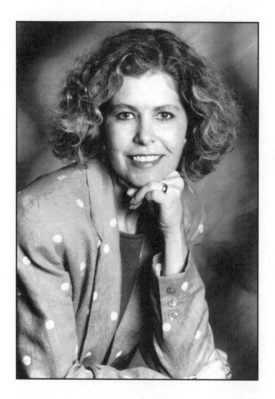

Karen Kaigler-Walker, Ph.D., is a professor of marketing and psychology at Woodbury University in Burbank,
CA who specializes in the relationship between women's
inner and outer selves. Formerly a consultant to the Texas
Governor's Commission on Aging, she has also served as
a delegate to a White House conference on older women.
She lives in Altadena, CA with her husband.